Live Cadaver

The True Story of Kellee Kendell and Scandalous Treachery Within the Medical Community

Phyllis Marks, JD
And Kellee Kendell

Second printing

Cover design courtesy of Denise Brilliant: Brilliantbox.co

ISBN: 069225711X

Printed in the United States of America

To William and Mary Marks, a thousand thanks
for coming to get me. — P.M.

To my precious mother, Marlene Dietrich Kendell,
thank you for loving me enough to keep me alive.
If I had only listened to your warning. — K.K.

To all the women who will read this and benefit
from it. — P.M. and K.K.

Contents

Acknowledgements

This book is the fulfillment of a commitment, by the authors, to impact the lives of women by providing undeniable proof of the importance of taking a proactive stance in their medical treatment. Their lives could depend on it.

Phyllis Marks especially wishes to acknowledge the following:

Alice Stevenson, my best friend and confidant, who contributed invaluable input by patiently reading and rereading the manuscript. Thanks so much for being there for me, once again, anytime, day or night.

Marnie Case, my sister who introduced me to the awesomeness of the written word by teaching me to read, and providing me with my first library card. Thank you for your unwavering support and belief in me as a writer.

Deborah Mumford, my sister who never doubted my ability to undertake difficult projects and emerge victorious. Thanks for setting the bar so high for me.

Ronald Appleton, my brother who taught me, early, how to fight and be strong in the world of men. I still haven't forgotten how you left me on that sidewalk because I was a girl!

Ernest Laster, my friend and colleague who started me on the path to solo practice. Your sage advice and practical wisdom sustained me for years to come. Thanks for believing in me enough to give me the opportunity to succeed.

Cynthia Samples, my friend who has always had the courage to be direct and forthright. Thanks for reading the manuscript and giving me your honest and valuable opinions.

Ivory Dorsey, whose willingness to discuss my ideas and strategies in reference to our book, resulted in powerful ideas and approaches. Though our friendship is short in quantity, it has been long in quality.

Harry and Sue Saye, who provided me with the opportunity for profound spiritual evolution. Thank you so much for your patience, support, and understanding during the final stages of the production of this book.

Kellee Kendell especially wishes to acknowledge the following:

To all the dedicated doctors who worked tirelessly, on numerous occasions, to save my life. I thank each and every one of you. I will always remember your kindness.

To Dr. Robin Newburn, thank you for hearing my cries for help.

To my dear friends, Janet Boykin, Deatra Harris, Denise Brilliant, Suzanne Faith Parks, Chavala Ware, Letra McCoy, Tiffani Sossei, and the Hesling and Missouri families. Thank you for loving me when I couldn't love me.

To my son, Kendell Bouquette, my father, Richard Merrill Kendell, my sister, Angela Kendell Pogue, Ron Pogue and my cousin, Scott Goggin. Through your endurance, each of you has claim to a piece of my heart.

To Phyllis Marks, my dear friend, thank you for your courage and your relentless pursuit of justice. I love you, my friend.

In loving memory of Angela Kendell Pogue, I would choose you again.

Introduction

In the spring of 2000 Kellee Kendell was diagnosed with multiple uterine fibroids.

Although she had fibroids, she did not have the complications with which some women suffer. She was not having excessive bleeding and she had no difficulty with her periods. Her only complaint was some slight pressure on her bladder that felt like a urinary tract infection. That cleared up by the time she went to see her gynecologist in May 2000.

Kellee's gynecologist recommended that she have a procedure called uterine fibroid embolization (UFE). It was the first time she heard of it. Since this procedure was unfamiliar to her, a red flag should have gone up, immediately. She should have been asking questions like crazy, but she did not, because she placed all her trust in her doctor. Her doctor told her that UFE would eliminate her fibroids permanently and that it was considered to be the miracle cure. He said it was a simple 24-hour outpatient procedure and that she would have to stay overnight for observation. This turned out to be disastrously wrong.

In this society, as women, we have been programmed to believe that doctors are skilled and trained people who always know what they are doing and have our best interests at heart.

The majority of the time this is true. Women are apt to follow their doctors' recommendations without question. However, this societal belief is amazing since the media have been full of instances where this has been proven to be erroneous. There is a long history of drugs and products being prescribed for women long *before* the proper research and testing trials have been thoroughly performed. Whether we are aware of it or not, we blindly accept the unknown long-term effects of these drugs when we take them, sometimes with catastrophic results. Why is it that, as a group, women continue to allow themselves to be exploited by the almighty dollar?

A very recent example of this exploitation is hormone replacement therapy (HRT). Women have been taking these drugs for years and years, although medical researchers have always had evidence that these drugs can cause cancer. When these drugs were first introduced, the long term effects were listed as "unknown". Another example of disastrous results for a product marketed to women is the silicone implants. We know how devastating these implants were for women in terms of the tremendous health problems they developed from the silicone. And they are trying to bring the silicone implants back!

Owning our responsibility as women, we made a personal decision that we would not be silent about what happened to Kellee. We decided that other women deserve to know about the terrible effects she experienced as a result of her UFE, and from not educating herself about this procedure. While UFEs have proven to be a successful alternative for some women, there are still a lot of unknowns and, especially, the long-term effects.

It is our hope that Kellee's story will help to convince the medical community that there is much research that still needs to be done about fibroids and the treatment options for them. A March 2001 report by the National Institute of Environmental Health Sciences (NIEHS) indicates that by their late 40s, more than 80 percent of black women and nearly 70 percent of white women had developed benign uterine fibroid tumors. That is an incredibly huge market.

As a result of what happened to Kellee, we strongly believe it is imperative that women be *fully* informed about this topic and any treatment options their doctors propose for them. For any malady women should take a proactive stance in their medical treatment, and do their own research so they can make informed decisions with their doctors. It never occurred to Kellee to do her own research or to get a second opinion. She paid dearly for not doing so. If she had done even a modicum of research on UFEs, she would have known it was *not* the right treatment for her. She would have known she was *not* the prime candidate, as she was told by her doctors.

It is our hope that Kellee's story will help save many other women from the UFE nightmare Kellee had to endure for three long tortuous years.

As women we must come to the realization that, if we cannot depend on society to protect us in a more diligent manner, we must learn to protect ourselves.

Phyllis Marks, JD
Kellee Kendell
Atlanta, Georgia
May, 2005

Never underestimate the power of the pen.
—*William Monroe Trotter*

Prologue

Ohio February 2002

The darkness of the soul can be so black that no amount of light can penetrate it. Fear can grip your heart so tightly that you can feel the breath of life being slowly squeezed from your body. Pain can reach such proportions that the torture of it propels you to plead with God to be merciful and grant you death. I had arrived at that point in my life.

It was déjà vu. Everything that happened when I was forced to have my emergency surgeries in November 2000 was now happening in February 2002. The pain attacking my body was so vicious I was convinced it was devised by demons that lived in the pit of a fiery hell. The vomit that spewed forth from my mouth came in vile green torrents. If someone had thought to video record it, they would have been paid handsomely by Hollywood for its use in the next exorcist movie. Special effects would have been unnecessary for this scene.

IVs were attached, once again, to my body, and I had been told they were going to have to insert the wretched nasogastric tube to control my vomiting. Mercifully, Dr. Olson had come quickly to my bedside and ordered immediate sedation. When I came to, he was standing over my bed gently rubbing my forehead.

Tears filled my eyes as I looked up at him with guilt.

"Are you mad at me?" I asked.

"Why would I be mad at you Kellee?" he asked.

"Because you warned me in September, if I didn't allow you to operate, this would happen," I sobbed.

"Kellee, you were so scared, and you had already been through so much," he said. "I don't blame you for not wanting surgery that might beget another surgery."

He continued to rub my forehead as I shed silent tears.

"I'm going to have to get a CT scan to confirm my suspicions," he said, knowing I would hate it.

I was too terrified to ask what his suspicions were. I did not want to know. My heart sank as I thought about the contrast medium I would have to drink in order for the CT scan to be performed. I knew if I tried to swallow it, I would start vomiting again, and that would make the insertion of the nasogastric tube imperative. As it turned out, Dr. Olson had to have me sedated for the test to be performed.

The next morning I woke up and discovered that the nasogastric tube had been inserted. My mother was at my bedside. She was waiting for Dr. Olson to come to the hospital to tell us the results of the CT scan.

When Dr. Olson arrived he got right to the point.

"Kellee," he said, "it's just as I suspected, you have a bowel obstruction, and we have to go in and operate."

My worst fears had come to pass. I turned my gaze down to my tightly clasped hands. When I raised my head, I looked straight into Dr. Olson's eyes and said, "If you get inside and you find that I'll have to live the rest of my life with a bag attached to my stomach, let me die." I meant it. I knew I had to have this surgery in order to live, but I would rather die than live with a colostomy.

Dr. Olson looked at me with compassion but did not respond. His touch on my forehead was soft before he turned and walked out of the room.

In my heart I did not believe I would survive this surgery anyway. The pain I'd suffered over the last five months had to mean things were really bad inside me. I had not forgotten Dr. Olson's grim predictions back in September. If his predictions were that bad then, five months later, if I was still having pain, things just had to be worse. But in the slim chance that I did make it, I wanted to make my requests clear. I looked up at my mother.

"I want you to call Phyllis Marks and tell her what happened," I said. "Tell her to please continue to fight my case even if I die."

My mother's face was full of love as she looked down at my face and into my tear-filled eyes. "I'll call Ms. Marks," was all she would say as she stroked my hair.

Still in denial I thought, but I understood. My mother would never concede that death was a possibility for me.

I settled back in the bed, resigned to my fate. I believed with all my heart that Ms. Marks would understand how I felt even if I died. I believed that she would not let death silence me and leave my story untold. I was comforted as I realized that she was my guardian angel sent by God to pick up my blood stained banner and carry it to victory for me, if necessary. Whether I was alive or dead, she was the chosen one to replace the strength I no longer had. God knew exactly what He was doing when He sent her into my life.

My sister arrived at the hospital and she and my mother stayed with me until I was taken into surgery. Kendell did not come because he could not face seeing me like this and, quite frankly, I was glad he was not here. He had been traumatized enough and I wanted to spare him this latest pain. I felt I had somehow failed him even if it had not been intentional. For almost two years he witnessed his wonderfully vibrant mother being steadily reduced to a mere shadow of what he remembered her to be for all of his life.

As I was being wheeled into the operating room, Angie and

my mother kissed me on my forehead and reiterated their love for me. I told them I loved them too. I looked longingly at them as I drank in every aspect of their precious faces. I wanted to carry a vivid memory of them into surgery in case I never saw them again.

In the operating room the mask was placed over my face. This time the anesthesia was not replaced with the smell of Tuscany. It was just as well because that scent represented a different form of betrayal and trust. It would not be befitting for that to be my last memory of my life here on earth. As the blackness began to overtake me, my mind was transported to Jamaica where I saw myself riding a jet ski just before sunset. In the next instant I was on the back of my friend's motorcycle riding up in the mountains, headed towards Ricks Café to conclude the evening cliff diving.

Jamaica....

I woke up in the recovery room. It slowly dawned on me that I was still alive. I was barely conscious. I couldn't feel anything but I was aware that tubes, IVs and machines, were attached to my body. I heard the sound of voices just outside my room. Although my vision was blurred, my hearing was oddly razor-sharp.

"What in the world happened to her?" a voice asked that I did not recognize.

"It was due to a botched up mess in Atlanta," the second voice replied. It was Dr. Olson.

Botched up mess? He never told me that although I had asked many times what happened to me. Before I could think about it anymore, I slipped back into darkness.

Chapter One

On Top of the World

"Geez! Where is the office building I'm looking for?" I fumed. My mother who was sitting next to me in the passenger seat of my car, did not bother to answer. She was visiting me from Ohio. She knew I was just letting off steam and any answer from her would only make my agitation worse. Gripping the steering wheel tightly with both hands, I leaned up close to the windshield and peered up at the office building in front of us. I was still not sure this was the building where Dr. Daniel Snyder's office was located. We had been riding around in the same general area for the last twenty minutes looking for his office.

The last thing I wanted to do today was fit a doctor's appointment into my already overburdened schedule. All I wanted to do was get this over with as quickly as possible so I could put it behind me and move on. Now, I could not find his office. I thought I'd copied the directions down correctly. Apparently, I had made a mistake somewhere because finding his office was not happening. I was in a parking lot and that was all I was sure of.

It was May 15, 2000. A perfect day for the new millennium.

Atlanta was so pretty in the springtime. Two months ago the dogwood trees had been in full bloom, lighting up Atlanta with effervescent shades of pinks and whites. Fluffy green leaves now replaced the beautiful blossoms, and the leaf-laden branches swayed placidly in the springtime breeze. It was a bright and sunny day and the temperature was a perfect seventy-five degrees. It was the kind of day that made you feel good just to be alive. This feeling was welcome, especially coming on the heels of my fiasco in Naples, Florida.

I was tempted to turn around and go back home. I was having so much trouble locating Dr. Snyder's office building maybe God was trying to tell me something. Maybe this was a bad omen. I was to learn later that I should have paid attention to these warnings instead of suppressing and ignoring them. As women, we are given gifts of intuition, and we should never ignore the quiet voices of warning that so often come to us.

Caught between my temptation to just forget it and go home and my paranoia about the masses that had been found in my abdomen, I was in a quandary. I began a mental dialogue with myself. Why should I bother with going to see this doctor when I'm feeling fine? The symptoms I had in Naples were all gone. This is just a waste of my time! I jerked the steering wheel sharply to the left in order to turn the car in the direction of home, but then immediately put my foot on the brake. I placed my head on the steering wheel as I tried to decide what to do. Then I sat up and looked out the window at the beautiful day, as I clenched my teeth in frustration.

Aggravated, I slammed my body into the back of the car seat. I was becoming more and more irritated. I was irritated because I was anxious to get back on track with my real estate investment career, and this was an unwelcome interruption. Making an abrupt and wide U-turn, I swung into a parking space and shoved the car into park. I twisted around in my seat until I was facing my mother, and then angrily folded my arms across my chest.

"Mommy!" I said in exasperation, "As you can see, I can't find Dr. Snyder's office and, quite frankly, I don't see the point in having to go to this appointment anyway when my urinary tract infection has cleared up. I think you're making a mountain out of a mole hill over these masses." I still called my mother "Mommy" even though I was 36-years-old. My verbal demeanor was resentful and it conveyed an unmistakable air of pouting and venting.

I had always resisted being told what to do, by anyone, and had been accused many times of being too aggressive and forward. Nevertheless, my spirited nature had served me well and gotten me far all of my life. Courageous and fearless, I had come to Atlanta ten years ago with $50 in my pocket. At that time, I had recently undergone open heart surgery and had to file bankruptcy due to all the medical bills that I would never be able to pay. My parents had a fit when I told them I was moving to Atlanta, but I'd stubbornly refused to change my mind. It seemed like such a long time ago.

My mother, who had been looking straight ahead ignoring my little temper tantrum, turned her head and was now looking sternly at me. "Kellee," she said with an attitude that brooked no compromise, "we've been through all this and I want you to get your cell phone out right now and call Dr. Snyder's office for the directions from where we are. Dr. Goodman called me in Ohio, from Naples, just to get your phone number so she could call you. She told you before you left Naples that you were supposed to get checked by a doctor when you got to Atlanta. That was almost two months ago. I don't think you should put it off any longer. Now, call Dr. Snyder's office."

Deliberately ignoring what my mother had just said, I blurted, "But I feel fine now! My urinary tract infection has cleared up! You know how doctors are. They're sure to find something from nothing if you give them half a chance!" Another tug from my intuition was asserting itself but I was allowing my emotions to overshadow this powerful hint that something was not right about all this, and deserved closer inspection.

"Kellee, what you're saying doesn't make sense, "she said, losing patience. "You'd better get that cell phone out right now and call Dr. Snyder's office. I mean it. You're being silly and you know it. Get on that phone and get the directions."

I stayed jammed up against the driver's side door and did not move. I knew it would be hard for me to ignore my mother's voice of reason, but I had no intention of giving in right away. I wanted the satisfaction of stewing in my soup and being rebellious for a little longer. I was having conflicting thoughts about what I should do, but I did not take the time to ask myself why I was feeling this way. I should have.

My mother looked over at me and sighed. She tried a different approach and said, "We can go shopping tomorrow when all this is over." She knew I loved shopping with her and was trying to cajole me into a better mood. Shopping together had been a lifetime tradition with us. Some of my friends chided me that I had never cut the umbilical cord with my mother. She has always been my best friend and champion supporter. She was stubbornly trying to look after my best interests now.

"Okay," I said, finally giving in, "I'll call Dr. Snyder's office." Besides, I knew I was not going to win this debate and I knew what my mother was saying was right. I should at least explore it. I was being obstinate and I knew it. Turning around and reaching for my purse on the back seat, I said, "I'll get the directions so I can get this over with but you'll see you're making a big fuss about nothing."

"I appreciate that, Kellee," she said, no longer conveying her air of steel and determination. She knew she had won and was being gracious about it. "On the way home we can decide to do something nice for dinner."

I dialed Dr. Snyder's office number and we were soon turned around heading in the right direction.

Ten minutes later we walked into the reception area of Dr.

Snyder's office. My mother immediately sat down in a chair, picked up a magazine and started flipping through the pages. I looked around and saw that, except for us, the reception area was empty. I found this to be odd as every other doctor I had contacted in an effort to get an appointment, had been booked up for months. Another bad omen. Some of them were not even taking new patients. Suddenly, I had a feeling of uneasiness. I shrugged it off. I would ask myself months later why I did not pay attention to these feelings of warning that were coming through so loud and clear.

Shaking off my feelings of apprehension, I walked up to the receptionist's window. The lady in the office area behind the window slid the window open, checked me in for my appointment time, and asked me if this was my first visit with Dr. Snyder. She looked professional in her white uniform and her blond hair was pulled neatly back away from her face in a bouncy ponytail. She was smiling and friendly as she told me to come to the door so she could take me back to Dr. Snyder's office. I thought this was really fast. Drive through doctor's service? No waiting at all. Big, big, warning sign that I ignored.

As I walked through the door, she stepped aside so I could come in. She said, "Kellee I'm Sheila, Dr. Snyder's nurse. Since this is your first visit with Dr. Snyder he'll want to talk with you before he examines you. We walked down the hall toward his office. As we passed by an examination room, she pointed and said, "When you're finished talking with the doctor, come back to this room and I'll get some basic information from you."

We entered Dr. Snyder's office and she said, "Kellee, have a seat and Dr. Snyder will be with you in a few minutes." I sat down and Sheila turned around and walked back down the hall.

As I sat in front of Dr. Snyder's desk, I looked around his office. My eyes were caught by the presence of a rather large and quite beautiful aquarium. The fish that swam around in it were brightly colored and very healthy looking. It was a well-cared for aquarium because the water looked clear and fresh. How unique, I thought. I had never seen an aquarium in a doctor's office before. There were the usual degrees and certificates on the wall but there was nothing usual about the aquarium. I smiled as I looked at the pleasant family pictures that were sitting on the credenza behind the desk.

There was a small square table next to my chair with some magazines on it. I picked up one of the magazines and began leafing through it. As I turned the pages, my mind began to wander back over the last eight months. Once these thoughts started surfacing, I lost my interest in reading. I tossed the magazine back on the table and sat back in my chair. I leaned my head against the back of the chair and closed my eyes. I was finally able to relax from my ordeal of trying to locate the office. My mind drifted back to Naples.

I had fled Atlanta eight months ago with Naples as my appointed destination. I was fed up with the daily rush hour traffic that I seemed to be stuck in all the time. I remember clearly the day I decided to flee. I was driving along Georgia 400, which is famous for its grid-locks during rush hour traffic. At that time, it seemed that the story of my life was to be stuck in traffic and I had grown weary of it. I was tired of fighting with ungrateful tenants who had no concept of what was appropriate behavior in a lease situation. The outrageous things they did to my rental property were beyond belief. I had begun to feel like I was on a treadmill that did not have a pause button. I was juggling a full time real estate investment career simultaneously with being a model and model's agent. I was so driven to be successful!

I had not stopped to catch my breath for ten years. I realized that I came to Atlanta ten years ago driven by the need to put as much distance as I could between myself and the man that had broken my heart into a million pieces. I loved the Tuscany cologne that he wore but I had needed to get the smell of it out of my nostrils. Ironically, that smell was to haunt me for years to come. Shifting in my chair, I was annoyed that I was thinking about Tuscany which would invariably start me to thinking about the most horrible emotional pain of my life. It had been hard for me to get over his betrayal of my trust and I could not stop viewing men with suspicion and disdain. I knew I had become cold and unfeeling when it came to relationships, but I could not help it.

I first noticed Mr. Tuscany as a young girl of seventeen while watching him play basketball as I sat upon the hill at Ohio Dominican College. I had fallen in love with him several years later. I was well into the relationship before I realized I had involved myself with someone who needed to validate his own identity by demeaning mine. Much later, I learned that our whole relationship was built on a tower of lies, and everyone seemed to know this but me. The truth was revealed in idle conversation with a friend and it was like, oops! I thought you knew. This discovery had done irreparable damage to my self-esteem and it became difficult to determine which was more painful: The knife in my back from the betrayal or the knot in the stomach from all the deception. A Hallmark card has never been written that could describe the extent of the pain that had devastated my emotions.

Although I had fled from Mr. Tuscany, I had numerous conversations with him over the years. I guess it was my way of trying to maintain a semblance of dignity by trying to prove to him that the separation from him had not stopped me one bit. I tried to apply super-glue to my broken heart but it was not mended. I was stripped of the ability to love, much less trust any other man. The risk of betrayal was too great and I could not come to terms with it. In the destruction of our relationship, he changed the rules and I was determined to never be vulnerable like that again. I began to take pride in knowing that my heart was cold and callous, beyond being touched by any man.

I forced myself to change my train of thoughts, and I nestled more comfortably in the chair. I thought fondly of my son Kendell who is the love of my life. A smile tugged at my lips when I remembered how excited we were when we arrived in Naples. We thought we had found paradise. Kendell was only 13 years old at the time and had been ecstatic about us going on another one of our exciting adventures. He was used to exciting things happening with me, so he did not question the abruptness of my move to Naples. When we arrived in Naples, we were so pleased with our paradise that we thought we would never have to go on a vacation again.

I found myself frowning as I remembered that Naples turned out to be a complete disaster for me. I had really been glad to get away from there. Just before leaving Naples, I developed what I thought was a urinary tract infection. Despite my drinking copious amounts of water and abstaining from coffee, the irritation still had not cleared up after a week. I had gone to see Dr. Goodman for a checkup and to get some medication for my discomfort. In the process of the examination, she felt what she described as "masses" in my lower pelvic area. She wanted me to get an ultrasound. Since I refused to allow anything to interfere with my planned escape from Naples, I promised her I would see a gynecologist once I arrived in Atlanta.

I did not take the time to think and analyze the fact that running from Naples would not fix my problems. I would still be there whenever I arrived at my next destination. It is impossible to run from yourself and, sometimes, you have to stand flat-footed and confront your worst demons. If you do not you will simply postpone this self-introspection for another day, because it is not going to go away. This should have been clearer to me as a result of my attempt to run from myself by relocating to Atlanta ten years ago.

Once in Atlanta I forgot about what Dr. Goodman had said. It was not until she called my mother in Ohio that I even thought about it again. My mother had been upset. "Kellee," she had asked, accusingly, "why is Dr. Goodman calling here looking for you? Did you go and get yourself checked out in Atlanta?" Recalling this conversation caused all the memories of Naples and its myriad problems to come flooding back. I did not like my thoughts but they persisted. I had been so lonely in Naples, and even my long distance relationship had not been enough to satisfy me. It lacked meaning anyway. Ever since Mr. Tuscany, I had developed a protective and hard shell around my heart and none of my relationships could touch me at my core. On top of all this, I had a bad job experience. Yes, I had become very unhappy in Naples.

Restlessly, I shifted in my chair and reached for another magazine. Before I could open it Dr. Snyder walked into the office. I stood up and was instantly struck by his boyish looks. He was not tall but he had a powerful presence. His eyes were a flashing bright brown and they seemed to have a twinkle of perpetual amusement in them. I was taken by his vibrant demeanor and I liked him immediately.

He walked toward me with his hand extended and said, "Kellee, I'm Dr. Snyder. I'm pleased to meet you." His grip was warm and friendly. He released my hand as I sat back down.

He sat down in the chair next to mine. How down to earth, I thought.

"I really like your aquarium, it's beautiful," I said, laughing. "I've never seen an aquarium in a doctor's office before."

He turned and looked at the aquarium, laughing too. "I know it's unusual but I really like aquariums and it gives me a sense of peace and serenity to have one in my office."

For the next twenty minutes we talked about everything under the sun that had to do with our children, and the extracurricular activities they were involved in. If he was trying to get me relaxed it was working. I really liked this doctor! I was thinking, this doctor is certainly willing to take the time to make his patients feel comfortable with him by giving them the opportunity to get to know a little bit about him. I was delighted.

Finally, he said, "So, what brings you in to my office today, Kellee?"

"As I mentioned, I just moved back to Atlanta from Naples.

Before I left Naples, I went to see Dr. Anna Goodman because I thought I had a urinary tract infection. When she examined me, she said she felt some masses in my abdomen. She did say the masses might be fibroids but she would not be able to make a diagnosis without an ultrasound. My mother's been really worried but I've felt fine since I've been back in Atlanta. I don't have any more urinary discomfort. My mother's attitude has made me a little paranoid, though. What do you think the masses could be?" I leaned toward Dr. Snyder, anxiously awaiting his answer.

He smiled at my intensity and said, "From what you're describing so far, I don't think you have anything to worry about. It sounds like you might have uterine fibroids. Fibroids are very common in African-American women. However, we need to be sure that's what the masses are. We'll probably need to do an ultrasound but I'll know more once I've examined you. Do you know what fibroids are?"

"I've heard of fibroids before but I don't really know a lot about them," I replied.

Dr. Snyder slouched into a more comfortable position and placed his hands on the back of his head. He said, "Fibroids are tumors that develop in the muscular wall of the uterus. Nobody knows exactly why they develop or why African-American women are more prone to get them. It's a possibility that they can become cancerous but it's not likely. Fibroids don't always cause symptoms. Their size and location can lead to problems for some women, including pain and heavy bleeding. Have you had any pain or heavy bleeding?"

"No," I answered, "I haven't had any problems with my periods and I'm not anemic. The only thing I've had is the urinary discomfort and that has cleared up. I'm not having any problems at all right now."

"That's good," Dr. Snyder said, continuing with his explanation. "Fibroids can range in size from very tiny to very large. If you do have fibroids it doesn't sound like they've become a problem for you."

I was visibly relieved as I asked, "So what do I need to do if I have fibroids?"

Dr. Snyder stood up and walked toward the door. He said, "Right now I'm going to take you back to the examination room where Sheila will help you get undressed. She'll get some basic background information from you and I'll come in when she's finished. Once I've examined you I'll be able to tell you what you need to do. Let's get you to the exam room." I followed him out of the office and down the hall.

Sheila met me outside the door of the examination room and led me over to the scales. She had the air of an efficient and pleasant person. Once she got my weight we walked back to the room, and she told me to sit on the table.

As I pushed myself up onto the table, I asked, "Should I get undressed?"

"Not right now," she said, as she lifted the blood pressure apparatus off a hook on the wall. "First I'll need to get your blood pressure and some other information since this is your first time seeing Dr. Snyder." She wrapped the blood pressure cuff around my arm, and placed the stethoscope in her ears as she started pumping the cuff. "Ninety-eight over sixty," she said as she pulled the stethoscope out of her ears and efficiently unwound the cuff from my arm.

Picking up a clipboard Sheila sat down on a chair and began to write information on the form that was clipped to it. She started asking me questions and had her pen poised to record my answers.

"Are you allergic to anything?"

"No."

"What is your height?"

"Five-ten."

"Your age?"

"Thirty-six."

"How many children do you have?"

"One."

"How many times have you been pregnant?"

"Once."

"Why is it that you need to see the doctor today?"

I took a deep breath as I prepared to give her the short version of my answer. I said, "Well, I'd been having some urinary discomfort. It felt like a urinary tract infection so I went to see Dr. Anna Goodman in Naples, Florida, and I got a checkup in late March. She gave me some medicine and it cleared up. While she was examining me, the doctor said she felt a mass in my abdomen and said I should get it checked out once I got to Atlanta. So that's why I'm here."

"Okay," she said, as she continued to write.

Once she stopped writing, Sheila looked up and asked, "Are you taking any medications?"

"No."

"When was your last menstrual period?"

"February 27, 2000."

"Was your last menstrual period normal?"

"Yes."

"How often do you have your period?"

"Every twenty-eight days."

"How long are your periods?"

"Four days."

We went through a series of other medical questions on the form and Sheila checked the appropriate boxes according to my answers.

When she completed all the questions, she stood up and said, "Okay, I've got your basic medical history for the doctor. You can get undressed now." She handed me a paper gown. "Put this gown on and I'll come back in a couple of minutes with Dr. Snyder."

It did not take me long to get undressed and, before long, both Sheila and Dr. Snyder were back in the room.

I have always hated pelvic examinations as I am sure most women do. It can be an uncomfortable and humiliating experience. However, Dr. Snyder was very gentle and talked as he performed his examination and this had a calming effect on me. As he palpated my uterus he said, "Yes, I can feel what appear to be several fibroids in your uterus. They feel like they're pretty large in size. I'm surprised you're not having any symptoms other than some slight pressure." As he removed the speculum and snapped off his rubber gloves, he said, "You can get dressed now. I want you to get an ultrasound so I can confirm my diagnosis of uterine fibroids. We're going to need to go to another location about ten miles from here to do the ultrasound. Sheila will give you the directions."

"What!" I exclaimed. "Where do I have to go? It's in the middle of rush hour! The last thing I want to do is to get stuck in rush hour traffic!'

"It's not really that bad, Kellee," Dr. Snyder said. "You'll be there before you know it and I really think you need to get an ultrasound so I can be sure we're dealing with fibroids. I'll meet you there." He opened the door and walked out of the room.

Exasperated, I looked at Sheila who was walking toward the door. Once at the door, she looked back, smiled and shrugged. She said, "It's better for you to get it over with than to have to come back. Besides, you'll know for sure that you have fibroids and you'll feel better. I'll meet you at the desk with directions on how to get there." She walked out of the room and closed the door behind her.

I was definitely not happy with this turn of events and I got dressed in a hurry. I got the directions, rushed my mother out of the office, and arrived at the other office building in a shorter time than I had anticipated. I was relieved about that. I was surprised to see that Dr. Snyder had followed us, so quickly, to the other location. He was already getting out of his car. He waved at us as he headed toward the building. This guy must be the most conscientious doctor in the world!

Once we were inside the building, my mother and I walked into the lobby of the second office. I was taken aback by what I saw. I looked at my mother out of the corner of my eye and I could see she was just as surprised as I was. She was looking around in amazement as she sat down and picked up a magazine.

The lobby was like something out of an old-time picture book. The room was decorated with numerous antiques and old-time sports memorabilia adorned the walls. I felt like I was in the middle of an old Spaghetti warehouse restaurant where the arrangements consisted of tables with rotating stirrups. In the midst of all the sports memorabilia were posters depicting the terms of pregnancy. I could not help chuckling to myself. The posters looked odd but it presented a sure reminder of where you really were.

As I sat down, I had to wonder what hockey sticks and football jerseys had to do with the most intimate parts of a woman's body. I looked over at my mother, who returned my look with raised eyebrows.

I had not sat long when the laboratory technician came and escorted me to the examination room where Dr. Snyder was waiting. He sat in the room during the whole time the technician was performing the ultrasound. He did everything but hold my hand! I remember thinking, I've either hit the mother lode in finding the most sincere and caring gynecologist in Atlanta or my condition is worse than I realized. This doctor was awesome.

I felt lucky when it came to doctors. For two years before my open heart surgery, I had faced numerous near-death experiences due to a ventricle septal defect. I felt that God smiled on me when I ended up having the top cardiologist and the top thoracic surgeon in the city. They both fought hard to repair the defect in my heart, and to give me the gift of normalcy through open heart surgery. Thanks to their obvious love for humanity and commitment to excellence in the pursuit of their practice of medicine, I was able to begin a normal life within two weeks after my surgery. They repaired the defect and I never again had one moment's problem with my heart.

I'm sure that my wonderful experience with my heart surgery doctors had a lot to do with my instantly developing the same feelings of trust with Dr. Snyder. I had experienced nothing but the best with doctors, and it never occurred to me that it could be any other way.

Finally, the ultrasound was completed. I got dressed and met with Dr. Snyder in an office that was in the same suite. He went over the results of the ultrasound with me.

"Well, Kellee," he said, "it's just as I suspected. You have multiple uterine fibroids. The size of your fibroids makes your uterus the size of an eighteen-week pregnancy."

I gasped in surprise and said, "But how could that be? My stomach is so flat!"

Dr. Snyder shook his head as he looked down at the printed results of my ultrasound. He said, "Well that's what the ultrasound results indicate. At some point, your fibroids could become a problem for you because of their size, and they might get larger."

Worried, I asked, "What can I do to get rid of them?" I was beginning to be disturbed by these little foreign entities that had invaded my body.

Dr. Snyder said, "The ideal way to get rid of fibroids is to have a hysterectomy."

"What!" I exclaimed. "If I had a hysterectomy I wouldn't be able to have children anymore, would I?"

"That's correct. Are you interested in having more children?" he asked.

"Absolutely!" I replied vehemently. "Although I'm not married now, I'm only thirty-six-years-old and I want to leave my options open. I only have one child. Plus, isn't the recovery time for a hysterectomy six weeks? I wouldn't have time right now for it even if I wanted it."

"There are other options for treating fibroids, though," he

said. "Two in particular I would recommend for you since you don't want a hysterectomy."

"You bet I don't want a hysterectomy," I said with finality. "We don't need to talk about that anymore because it's definitely not an option I would consider. I want to keep my uterus and keep my options open for having children in the future. What are the options you would recommend?" I asked, as I braced myself for an unpleasant answer.

Smiling at the expression on my face, Dr. Snyder said, "It's actually not that bad. The first option is a shot called Depo Lupron. The shot will have the effect of shrinking your fibroids. It will stop your period and you will experience menopausal like symptoms. You'll have mood swings, hot flashes, and night sweats. The second option works in conjunction with the shot and it's called a myomectomy. That's where I would go in and surgically remove the fibroids from the uterus. Once the shot has shrunk the fibroids then myomectomy might work for you."

"How long do you think I would need to take the shot?" I asked, interrupting his narration.

"Well, that depends," he answered. "I would start you off with a ninety-day dose, and then we would see if your fibroids shrink during the ninety-day period. You would come back in ninety days so I can see how you're doing. It's up to you if you want to take the shot. Given your busy lifestyle and desire to preserve your fertility, I think this option would work best for you, although the shot is temporary. It will at least give you the time to think about what you might want to do in the future, and to see how much your fibroids shrink."

"Okay!" I said, dramatically bringing my hands together and clasping them. "This sounds like the right treatment for me. It fits in with my busy schedule because I really don't have time to be sick and incapacitated. I'll take the ninety-day Depo Lupron shot."

Dr. Snyder left the room and returned with the shot. He said, "I'm sorry Kellee, but I'm going to have to give you the thirty-day injection. I just discovered we're out of the ninety-day injections. It just means you'll have to come back in thirty days for your next injection, but that won't be all bad. We can see how you're doing and if your fibroids have shrunk at all."

After my shot, I was anxious to get out of there. I was pleased with my appointment with Dr. Snyder. He sent me on my way with instructions on what to do if I experienced any problems. My mother was relieved when I told her the masses turned out to be fibroids. I had such good feelings about Dr. Snyder. I felt, once again, I have found a doctor I can trust and one that really cares about me. It cannot get any better than that.

I got in my car feeling on top of the world. I was relieved to have this little episode behind me. Now, I could get on with getting my real estate investment career back on track with full speed ahead.

Once in the car, I talked excitedly with my mother about all my plans. Already, my thoughts were flying with ideas on how I could best take my real estate investment career to the next level. It was only up from here!

Little did I know that the next day's events would start me on a path leading to three long tortuous years of hell.

Chapter Two

The Prime Candidate

The next day dawned sunny and bright. It was another beautiful day in Atlanta. I yawned and had a wonderful stretch as I pulled the covers more tightly up to my chin. I could hear my mother downstairs rattling around in the kitchen. I rolled over and glanced at the clock. It was almost six-thirty. Reluctantly, I crawled out of bed to go and wake Kendell so he could get ready for school. I always got up with Kendell even though I knew he was old enough now to get ready by himself.

As I sat on the side of the bed, I thought about how hard it had been for me to fall asleep last night. My mind had been busy assessing my priorities and deciding what my next real estate career endeavors would be. Now that I knew that my abdominal masses were nothing more than fibroids, I could put them on the back burner for now. I felt confident that the shot I received at the doctor's office yesterday would shrink my fibroids and make them nonexistent.

I got up, pulled my robe on, and padded over to Kendell's room. As I expected, he was still sound asleep. I smiled as I stood inside the doorway looking at how deeply he had managed to burrow under the covers.

"Kendell," I called, "it's time for you to get up and get ready for school. Mimi is downstairs fixing you some breakfast."

His muffled answer under the covers, assured me he would be getting up in just a minute.

As I walked back to my room, I started thinking about the day and all I would accomplish. I marveled at what a difference a day could make. I was happy to be back in Atlanta and it truly felt like a new beginning. I smiled as I thought about it. A fresh start, in a brand new millennium. Who could ask for anything more? I was pleased to recognize that the same fire I had upon arriving in Atlanta ten years ago, was burning brightly today. Only this time, I saw a brighter future because I did not have any emotional baggage. The smell of Tuscany had receded deeply into the recesses of my memory. I was looking forward to starting the day shopping with my mother and then we would have lunch. It was a tradition we had maintained for as long as I could remember and I loved it.

I took my time getting ready for the day. I took a long and leisurely bath, luxuriating in the hot water as I soothingly sluiced the water over my body. The steam from the running water filled the bathroom, making it feel like I was in a steam bath at one of the local health clubs. After a while I reluctantly stepped out of the tub, and wrapped myself in an over-sized thick towel. It felt wonderful.

Walking into my bedroom to get dressed, I could hear my mother and Kendell squabbling downstairs in the kitchen. As I ruffled the towel through my still-damp hair, I smiled in amusement as I thought about how obsessed my mother was with nutrition. Skipping breakfast, or any meal for that matter, was not an option for her. She was obsessive about her children and grandchildren eating healthfully. For some reason Kendell liked to push her buttons on this point, and assert what he thought was his right to not eat breakfast if he didn't want to. Oh well, I thought, they'll work it out.

I got dressed and went downstairs. As I entered the kitchen, my mother was sitting at the table watching Kendell who sat eating his breakfast with an obvious air of resentment. I could tell he could not wait to get out of there. He loved his Mimi dearly, but he was at the age where he did not like being fawned over. He did not understand why Mimi felt the need to do this and he was all righteous indignation.

Kendell looked up and said, "Hi, Mom," as he gulped down his last spoonful of oatmeal. Having finished, he bolted from the table and headed for the sink to rinse out his bowl. With relief that that ordeal was over, he hurried into the foyer and retrieved his book bag. Following, I said, "Kendell, do you have everything you need? Don't forget anything because I don't want to have to come to the school to bring anything to you. Mommy and I are going shopping today."

Kendell looked at me with mischief in his extraordinary green eyes. "Of course not Mom," he said, as he smirked at me. "I wouldn't want to interfere with your shopping." Before I could respond he dashed out the door.

I followed Kendell outside and watched him walk down the street to where the school bus would pick him up. I still could not get over how quickly he had grown up. Where had all the years gone? He had grown into a tall and handsome young man and in another four years, he would be going off to college. I felt a poignant lump of sadness in my throat as I turned and walked back into the house.

By the time I came back into the house, my mother was sitting out on the patio enjoying her habitual cup of coffee. She was looking out at the beautiful trees that lined the back of my property. She was already dressed and ready to go. As I looked at my mother, I marveled at how beautiful she still was. Marlene Dietrich Kendell was a real class act. Her bright silver hair was cut stylishly short and not a hair was out of place. No matter what she was wearing, she always looked like she'd just stepped out of a fashion magazine. Today she was wearing an elegant black pant suit with a vibrant turquoise blue silk blouse. She exuded class and style from the top of her neatly coiffed hair, down to the bottoms of her perfectly manicured feet. I only hoped I would look as good when I had a teenaged grandchild.

I always knew I was blessed to have such a wonderful mother. My mother was not just beautiful on the outside, but she had such a sweet demeanor. All her friends and relatives adored her. She was deeply spiritual and would not hesitate to lend a helping hand if it was needed. Her devotion to my sister and I was something we both treasured.

I leaned over and hugged her as I said, "It's a good morning Mommy. How are you feeling today?"

"I'm fine, Kellee," she smiled. "How's my girl?"

We sat and talked as she drank her cup of coffee and I ate my breakfast. We were in no hurry. Besides, the stores were not open yet. My mother always enjoyed listening to the exuberance in my voice as I went into intricate detail about how I was going to do this or that. She loved my energy and the enthusiasm with which I tackled every aspect of my life. She felt like she was on an adventure when she came to visit me. We always had a lot to catch up on. I was her exciting little baby girl and it was fun for her to live vicariously through me.

Around nine-thirty we left to begin our day of fun.

We had a wonderful day of shopping. We ate at one of our favorite places for lunch, and I chattered non-stop the whole the time we were eating. I had her laughing at the stories I told her about my challenges in Naples. It really was funny in retrospect.

I was to remember that fantastic day with my mother for a long time. It was the last day we would have together doing all the things we loved to do, before my life was to change, forever.

We came home weighted down with the packages from all the bargains we could not resist taking advantage of. We arrived just in time to be there before Kendell got home from school. We had so many packages that we had to maneuver to get through the door. We dropped our bags on the floor, and then my mother plopped down on the couch in sheer exhaustion.

I ran upstairs to my bedroom to check my messages and as I entered the room, the phone rang.

I reached for the receiver, picked it up and said, "Hello?"

"Hello, Kellee?" It was Dr. Snyder.

"Yes, this is Kellee," I answered with surprise. "Dr. Snyder," I asked, "is everything alright?"

"Oh, yes," he hastily responded, "everything is fine. I didn't mean to scare you. Actually, I was calling to tell you some good news."

"Really," I said with obvious relief.

"I discussed your case with a colleague of mine," he said. "There is a procedure called uterine fibroid embolization and he tells me you are the prime candidate for it."

"What did you say it was?" I asked. It sounded like Greek to me and I had never heard of it before. Of course I didn't really know that much about fibroids until yesterday.

"Uterine fibroid embolization," he repeated. "It's called UFE for short and this is a procedure that permanently gets rid of fibroids. It's a simple 24-hour outpatient procedure. I talked with Dr. Paul Langford about your case and he is the doctor that performs UFEs. What they do is insert a tube through your groin and shoot polyvinyl alcohol particles into your uterine arteries. This has the effect of blocking the flow of blood to the fibroids, which will cause them to die. They will simply disintegrate and dissolve out of your system. The whole procedure takes thirty to forty-five minutes."

I was wondering why Dr. Snyder did not tell me about this yesterday.

"But I thought we were going to try the Depo Lupron therapy and see how that works," I said. "I just had the shot yesterday. I thought you said the *shot* would shrink my fibroids."

"The Depo Lupron will cause your fibroids to shrink," he said, "but, as I told you yesterday, this is only a temporary solution. UFE is a permanent solution."

"But I've already had the shot. Won't that interfere with the UFE?" I asked.

"Oh, no," he said, "I discussed that with Dr. Langford and he said Depo Lupron would not interfere. As I said, the difference between the shot and UFE is that one is temporary and the other is permanent. If your fibroids get any bigger, they could start to cause you problems. And in most cases, the fibroids do continue to get larger. If that happens, you might be forced to have a hysterectomy, and I know you don't want that. In discussing all this with Dr. Langford, he thought you would be a prime candidate."

"Well," I said, "I sure don't want to be faced with having to have a hysterectomy. So you think this procedure is the best treatment and would get rid of my fibroids permanently?"

"Absolutely," Dr. Snyder responded, "this way you can avoid having to have a hysterectomy."

"Okay, I'll do it if you recommend it," I said. "What do I need to do now?" If something this simple would permanently get rid of my fibroids, I was all for it.

"You need to call Dr. Langford who is an interventional radiologist. He's the colleague that I spoke to. In fact, he's expecting your call." We discussed UFE a little more and then Dr. Snyder gave me the phone number to call. Then we hung up.

I ran downstairs to tell my mother about Dr. Snyder's conversation. I sat down on the couch next to her.

"Well, Mommy," I said, "that was Dr. Snyder who just called me, and he was telling me about this procedure called a uterine fibroid embolization. It's called UFE for short. It's a simple 24-hour outpatient procedure and it gets rid of the fibroids permanently. They go in through your groin area and shoot some polyvinyl alcohol particles up into the uterine arteries. This blocks the blood flow to the uterus and causes the fibroids to die and dissolve out of your system." I said all this quickly hoping that it would impress her and win her support.

No such luck.

"I don't like the sound of it at all," she said. "It sounds like surgery to me. If it's so good why didn't Dr. Snyder tell you about it yesterday? Why would he give you a shot to shrink your fibroids and then call you back the next day to tell you about a procedure that gets rid of them permanently? There's something not right about that."

"Oh, Mommy, you're always worrying about every little thing," I said, exasperated. "If Dr. Snyder didn't think it was good for me, why would he recommend it for me?"

"I don't know," she responded. "Why did he recommend it?"

"Because he knows I don't want a hysterectomy and the UFE can get rid of my fibroids permanently," I replied. "What's so hard to understand about that?"

"What's hard for me to understand is why Dr. Snyder would give you a shot and then recommend you for something else the very next day," she said. "You're not even having any problems with your fibroids so why would you need this procedure?"

"My fibroids can get bigger and begin to give me problems," I said. "Besides, the shot will only shrink my fibroids temporarily. UFE gets rid of them permanently. Why are you being so difficult about this?"

"Because I have a bad feeling about this, Kellee," she said quietly.

"Oh, Mommy," I said with beginning irritation, "here we go again with the paranoia and the doom and gloom! You were so worried about the masses they found in my abdomen and that turned out to be nothing more than fibroids! Dr. Snyder knows I have had previous heart surgery and he wouldn't recommend me for a surgery that would be harmful to me. Can't you see that?"

"Why don't you give the shot a chance to work, Kellee?" Mommy asked, pleading. "What can that hurt?"

"Because Dr. Snyder said that the UFE is the best procedure for me and having the shot doesn't matter!" I exclaimed, heatedly. "After all, he's the expert and he knows what the best treatment would be. It was very conscientious of him to call me at home to tell me about it. This procedure will get rid of my fibroids permanently."

"But what about your trip to King's Island?" she asked. She was reminding me that Kendell and I would be leaving for our trip to Ohio next week where we were going to celebrate my nephew's birthday.

"That won't be any problem," I said, still trying to persuade her it was the right thing for me to do. "I'll see if I can have my UFE on Friday and I can go back to work on Monday. From what Dr. Snyder said, I'll only have a couple of days of discomfort and then I'll be fine. We're not leaving for Kings Island until later in the week."

"Nothing you say can convince me that what you're considering makes any sense," she said, stubbornly.

Exasperated, I got up and went back upstairs to my bedroom and sat on my bed next to the phone. I grabbed the receiver and dialed the number Dr. Snyder had given me to Dr. Langford's office. I could hear the phone ringing.

"Westside Radiology," a voice answered on the other end of the line.

"May I speak with Dr. Paul Langford?" I asked.

"May I ask what this call is in reference to please?" she asked.

"Yes," I said, "my name is Kellee Kendell and I was referred to Dr. Langford by my gynecologist, Dr. Snyder. I'm supposed to call Dr. Langford and talk to him about having a UFE done."

"Just a moment Ms. Kendell, I'll get Dr. Langford on the line," she said and placed me on hold.

A few seconds passed and a voice came on the line and said, "Hello, Ms. Kendell?"

"Yes," I responded.

"I'm Dr. Paul Langford," he said. "I've been expecting your call. I talked with Dr. Snyder earlier today about your case. I understand you're interested in having a UFE?"

"Well, I think I am," I said. "Dr. Snyder told me that you

perform UFEs. He said you thought I was the prime candidate for this procedure."

"Yes, from what he tells me you are. UFEs are perfect for women with your medical history," he said. Then he went on to repeat, almost verbatim, everything Dr. Snyder had said about UFEs.

After he finished, I asked, "How long would I have to stay in the hospital?"

"It's a simple 24-hour outpatient procedure," Dr. Langford answered. "We keep you in the hospital overnight for observation. You will experience some discomfort for a couple of days, but it will clear up after that and you can go back to work."

"Wow," I said, genuinely impressed, "this sounds like a miracle." If I could get rid of my fibroids with only two days down time, that would be absolutely great. "So what do I need to do now?" I asked.

"All we need to do is schedule a time for you to have your UFE," he answered.

"Well, I'd like to get it done as quickly as possible," I said. "If I got it done on a Friday, could I go back to work by Monday?"

"Yes, that would be no problem," he replied. "As I said, it's a simple 24-hour outpatient procedure."

I was thinking about how convenient it would be to get it done over the weekend. Then, I could hit the ground running on Monday. Also, my mother was here and would be here in case I needed her during my two-day recuperation period.

"Can I get my UFE scheduled for this Friday at Butler Hospital?" I asked. "I live right around the corner from there."

"I can do it Friday but not at Butler Hospital," he replied. "I'm scheduled to be at Hillside Hospital on Friday, so if you can come to that hospital, I can do it."

"That wouldn't be a problem," I said. "Although I live closer to Butler Hospital, I can come to Hillside where you're scheduled to be. I want you to perform the UFE because Dr.

Snyder referred you. So when do I need to come to your office for a work up?"

"Oh, no," he quickly replied, "that won't be necessary. It's just a simple 24-hour outpatient procedure. We'll schedule a time and I'll meet you at the hospital."

"Okay, I'm ready to set it up," I said.

"I'll get my receptionist back on the line and she'll set up your UFE appointment," he said. "She'll also get your insurance information and get your medical records faxed from Dr. Snyder's office. I look forward to meeting you at the hospital, Ms. Kendell. Hold on while I transfer you to Sarah."

Sarah came back on the line and I gave her all my insurance information. She scheduled my UFE for 2:00 p.m. on Friday at Hillside Hospital with Dr. Langford. She gave me instructions to not eat anything on the day of my procedure. I hung up the phone.

I went back downstairs and told my mother I had scheduled the UFE to be done on Friday. We picked right up where we left off after I finished talking with Dr. Snyder. She was still strongly opposed to my getting a UFE.

We were still going back and forth when Kendell got home. I was relieved for this interruption in our argument.

For the next two days, my mother begged and pleaded with me not to have the UFE. I got tired of arguing with her, but I was determined to have it done so I could get rid of my fibroids permanently. I knew she meant well, but I thought she was just being an overly protective mother. I was convinced that Dr. Snyder was the expert and I should do what he recommended. I trusted him and believed that if he referred me to Dr. Langford, he must be an excellent doctor too.

My mother was still pleading with me not to have the UFE when I walked out of the door on Friday, May 19th for my two o'clock appointment. It was late morning and I was to arrive at the hospital by twelve o'clock. I was hungry from not eating all day. I was anxious to get it over with so I could eat.

As I drove off, I waved cheerily at my mother, believing she would, once again, find that she had worried for nothing.

How wrong I turned out to be.

It was the last time my mother would see me as the healthy, vibrant, and enthusiastic little girl she had always known.

Chapter Three

A Simple 24 Hour Outpatient Procedure

It was May 19, 2000. I arrived at Hillside Hospital a little before noon and parked my car in the visitor's parking lot. I was looking forward to getting my UFE over with and being rid of my fibroids, forever.

I walked into the hospital and checked in at the outpatient department as I was instructed to do. The admitting clerk told me to have a seat in the waiting area and that the nurse would be out to get me shortly.

At 12:40 p.m., a stout looking nurse with a chart and a clipboard appeared through a door and called my name.

"Kellee Kendell," she said.

"Yes," I said rising from my chair.

"Kellee, come with me please," she instructed.

As I walked through the door, she said, "My name is Donna. I'm the R.N. that will be getting you ready for your UFE. I'll need to get some information from you so why don't you follow me."

I followed Donna to what looked very much like an emergency department. It was a large open area with several beds that were separated by long curtains that could be pulled around the bed for privacy.

"You can put your bags over there," she said, pointing to an empty chair that sat close to the bed. I put my things down on the chair.

"Why don't you get completely undressed, put on the gown, and then I'll come back and get some information from you," she said. She pulled the curtains along their tracks until my area was completely enclosed. She peeped around the curtain and said, "I'll be right back."

I undressed and sat on the bed waiting for Donna to return. It was not long before I heard her pulling the curtains aside to enter my area.

She got right into asking me background questions.

"Okay, Kellee, what is the reason for your admission?" she asked.

"Well, I'm here to get my fibroids zapped," I replied. "I have to stay overnight for observation and then I go home."

Donna was all efficiency as she took my vital signs and recorded my medical history on a form attached to the clipboard. When she finished, I looked at my watch and saw that it was 1:05 p.m. Less than an hour, I thought, and I'll be going for my UFE.

Donna was saying, "I'll need to get some blood from you so we can get the labs that need to be done before your procedure." She turned and picked up what appeared to be a plastic two-sided square basket. It had oodles of glass tubes in it with syringes, cotton balls and Band-Aids, and a myriad of other blood-work supplies. She plucked a long thin piece of rubber out of the basket, wrapped it tightly around my arm, and then secured it. She picked up a long huge-looking needle. I shuddered. I hated to get my blood drawn.

"Relax," she said, as she deftly swabbed the inside of my arm with alcohol, looking for a vein. Once she located it, she expertly slid the point of the needle in. She pulled the rubber tie loose as my blood spurted into the glass tube. I watched as my blood filled up two of the glass tubes.

Once Donna was finished she pressed the needle prick firmly with a cotton ball. She put a Band-Aid over the cotton ball and said, "Okay, Kellee, now you're all set for a while until they come and get you to take you to the radiology suite. Just before they come, I'll come back, get your I.V. started, and give you a shot that will relax you."

"Do you know how long that will be?" I asked. "I hope it won't be long because I'm really getting hungry. I haven't had anything to eat all day."

Looking at her watch, Donna replied, "It shouldn't be too much longer. Your procedure is scheduled for two o'clock and its 1:15 now." Picking up the basket, she said, "I'll call the nurse on 3 South with your lab results. If you need anything, just press the call button." She pushed the curtains aside and was gone.

I settled down in the bed and got more comfortable. I lay listening to the sounds of the hospital and the voices I heard as people walked around outside my curtained area. By two o'clock, still, no one had come. I must have fallen asleep because I awoke with a start and glanced at my watch. It was three o'clock. My stomach was really growling now. I was starving. I reached over and pressed the call button.

In a short time, I heard the curtains being pulled back and a different nurse appeared. "Hi, Kellee, my name is Cynthia," she said. " The shift has changed and I'll be taking care of you now. How can I help you?"

"I must have fallen asleep," I said. "I was supposed to have a UFE at two o'clock and it's now after three o'clock. Is Dr. Langford here yet? I haven't eaten anything all day and I'm starving."

"I'm not sure what's going on, I just got here," she answered. "I'll go and check on your status and I'll come back in a few minutes. Can I get you some ice chips or more water?"

"No," I replied. "Just please find out what's taking so long. I'm starting to feel weak from not eating."

"Okay, I'll be right back," she said, and left.

I reached over to the chair and retrieved my purse. I scrounged around inside for my cell phone. I pulled it out, flipped it open, and punched in my home number.

My mother answered the phone. "Hello?" she said.

"Hi Mommy, it's me," I said. "I just called to check on Kendell and let you know I'm alright."

"Have you finished already?" she asked. "That was really fast."

"Oh, no, I haven't even had my UFE done yet," I said, sounding dejected.

"What!" she exclaimed. "I thought your procedure was scheduled for two o'clock."

"It was," I said. "I guess they must be running behind schedule or something because they haven't come to get me yet. I haven't seen Dr. Langford."

"Kellee," she said, "this is a sure sign that you need to run for the door. You need to get out of there as fast as you can."

"There you go again," I said. "Please don't start on me about this. I've made up my mind that I'm going to get this done. Dr. Snyder said I'm the prime candidate for it."

"Kellee," she said, pleading, "God is giving you one last chance to get out of there. Honey, please come home."

"I wish you wouldn't carry on like this," I said. "You act like I'm getting ready to have some kind of major surgery. I've told you over and over, this is just a simple 24-hour outpatient procedure. I'll be home the first thing tomorrow morning."

"Kellee," she said in a rush, "I have such bad feelings about this. It just doesn't make sense to me. If you go through with this, I feel like something bad is going to happen to you."

I was relieved to look up and see the nurse coming back in the room. I used this as an excuse to get off the phone. "I've really got to go now," I said. "The nurse has come to give me my shot. I'll call you as soon as I'm finished. Bye, now." I flipped the cell phone closed before she could say anything more.

"Okay, Kellee," Cynthia said, "it's looks like they'll be

coming for you pretty soon. I'm going to start your IV and give you a sedative that will relax you for your procedure."

I stretched out my arm, and she took my arm with both hands, looking intently for a good IV site. She got my IV started without any problem. She took out a syringe and pulled the plastic cover off the top of the needle. She said, "I'm going to inject the sedative directly into your IV and you'll start feeling relaxed."

I watched as Cynthia inserted the needle in the tube connected to my IV and pushed the plunger down. Within a few seconds I began to feel very lightheaded.

That was my last memory of my life as Kellee Kendell before my UFE.

Sometime much later, I awakened feeling like someone had stuffed cotton balls in my mouth and my tongue felt thick. My mouth was parched and dry. I tried to swallow but I didn't seem to have enough saliva to perform this usually simple function. I felt lightheaded. I had no sense of time, and I had no idea whether it was day or night. I was having trouble remembering where I was. I could see I no longer had curtains around my bed and that I was in a regular hospital room. How had I gotten here?

Suddenly, my mind was slammed with the panicked awareness of the most excruciating pain I had ever felt in my life. It was centered in my pelvic region. It felt like someone was ruthlessly drilling a white-hot enormous screwdriver right through the center of my pelvis, and madly pushing it out through my back. Hot tendrils of pain licked up and down the backs and insides of my thighs, and across my stomach. Shocked by the intensity of the pain, I jerked upright in the bed. That was a mistake. I instantly became so nauseous I knew I was going to throw up. Gagging, I fell back on the bed and frantically hit the call button for the nurse. She responded at once and was standing at the foot of my bed within seconds.

"What has happened to me?" I asked in a muffled voice caused by the dryness of my mouth and throat. I did not recognize my voice. I was speaking softly because I was still afraid I would throw up. "What day is this? What time is it?"

"Today is Saturday and it's nine o'clock in the morning," she said. "You will not be leaving the hospital today due to your fever and vomiting," she said. She spoke in a matter-of-fact tone. There was no compassion in her voice and she struck me as being very cold and uncaring.

"Why am I having so much pain?" I asked weakly, trying to feel cautiously under the covers for the source of my tremendous pain.

"Don't you remember?" she asked. "You had a UFE yesterday." She was looking at me strangely.

"I know that," I said, "but nobody told me I would have this kind of pain." My breath was coming in short painful gasps due to the sharp pains that were firing through my stomach. Any attempt at movement made the pains sharper.

"Well, that's why you've got a PCA pump attached to your bed," she said as though I should have known this. "It has Morphine and you're supposed to push the button as needed."

I was beginning to believe I had awakened in hell. Was this nurse out of her mind? To control this terrifying pain, she would need to tape my index finger permanently to the push-button on the pump. This pain was to hell and gone from the mild discomfort I was told I would experience by Dr. Snyder and Dr. Langford. Where was Dr. Langford? In the midst of this thought, I pressed hard on the button to the PCA pump and felt immediate relief. The room began to blur and I drifted slowly into darkness.

I drifted in and out of awareness. It was as though I was watching myself from a foggy distance and I could not see clearly. Each time my head cleared from the Morphine, the pain would come back with cruel intensity. Unable to bear it, I would push the button on the pump and my mind would drift off into oblivion, once again.

During these intervals, I was aware that I felt feverish and unbelievably nauseous. I had several episodes of vomiting that I was powerless to control. More often than not, it was just dry heaves because I had nothing in my stomach to vomit. I remember thinking something must be horribly wrong. This pain is nowhere close to the description of what I was told I would experience after my UFE. Nothing had been said about vomiting and fever. Does Dr. Langford know about my condition? Why is he not here? I felt a raw fear starting to lick at my consciousness.

The next time I awakened, I was immediately assaulted with the most dreadful itching all over my body that anyone could imagine. I was nauseous and I vomited uncontrollably into an emesis basin that was kept at my bedside table. I could not scratch fast enough to give myself relief. The more I scratched the more intensely I itched. I thought maybe something on the sheets was making me itch like this. I hit the call button for the nurse.

Within seconds she appeared in the doorway.

"What is it that you need, Ms. Kendell?" she asked, walking up to my bed.

"I'm having the most terrible itching and it's about to drive me crazy," I answered, as I frantically scratched at my arms. "I keep throwing up. Why do I keep throwing up?" I was afraid to try to reach other parts of my body because too much movement would cause my pain to intensify. "Why isn't my doctor here helping me?" I asked.

The nurse did not answer. She walked around my bed and stood looking at my PCA pump.

"I want the sheets on my bed changed," I said. I thought maybe the sheets had something to do with the excessive itching and I was desperate to get them away from my body.

"Okay, but I don't think that's going to make a difference," she replied. "I'll go and get clean sheets and I'll be back in a few minutes."

I was still scratching as she walked out of the room. I was still scratching when she walked back into the room with the sheets cradled in her arms.

Changing the sheets turned out to be an ordeal. I had to turn over for the nurse to pull the sheets off the bed. The pain caused by this movement brought tears to my eyes. I could not stand for her to touch my body. It seemed as though my every nerve ending was primed for the sole purpose of conducting pain and itching to every far corner of my being. The nurse finally managed to get the bed changed and I settled down in the bed, completely exhausted.

I could not bear the itching and the pain any longer so I pressed the button on the Morphine pump. I felt the pump was the only friend I had in this nightmare place. I floated blessedly into a drug-induced stupor and then suddenly plunged into welcome darkness.

I did not awaken until the next morning. It was Sunday, May 21st. I was still in pain and I was still itching. My body was raw in several places from my uncontrollable scratching. I began to cry. How could I be this sick and no doctor come to see me? I was seeing objects that were not there and I was sure this was due to being on the Morphine Pump for two days. I wanted to go home where my mother could make me well again. I was afraid of what was happening to me.

I crawled carefully out of the bed, trying to avoid any abrupt movement that would incite another attack of itching and pain. I stood up slowly and leaned against the bed. It seemed that the pain had backed off a bit, but I knew it was still there lurking cruelly in the background. I decided I would get dressed and go home. What was the point of being here anyway if there was no doctor here to stop me? Has there ever been a doctor here to see me? I picked up my slacks, sat down on the bedside chair, and cautiously began to pull them on. Once I got my pants on, I stood up and managed to get everything on except my blouse.

The IV was in the way. I sat back down in the chair and pressed the call button for the nurse to come.

When the nurse entered the room, she looked surprised to see me sitting in the chair almost fully dressed.

"Ms. Kendell, what are you doing out of bed?" she asked.

"I'm going home," I said. "I need you to take this IV out of my arm so I can put my blouse on."

"You can't go home yet, Ms. Kendell, your doctor isn't available to discharge you," she said. "Besides, there's still too much Morphine in your body for you to be able to drive."

"I want to go home," I sobbed, trying to wipe the tears from my face. "Please, I want to go home."

"I'm sure the doctor will discharge you as soon as he gets here," she said kindly. "Why don't you get back in the bed until he comes? I'll disconnect your IV now but you'll have to wait for the doctor."

I was still crying as the nurse helped me back into bed. I thought, I've been abandoned by my doctor and left to suffer alone.

I drifted off to sleep and did not awaken again for several hours. When I woke up, I looked at my watch and I saw that it was after three o'clock. I began to get angry. I reached over and pushed the call button for the nurse. This was getting ridiculous. I had been waiting all day for Dr. Langford to come and discharge me, and he still had not shown up.

When the nurse appeared, I asked, "Has my doctor come to discharge me yet? I want to go home."

"No, Ms. Kendell," she replied, "but we did put a call into your doctor. He'll probably be here any minute now."

"I don't care if he's not here," I said angrily. "I'm going home right now. I've been waiting here all day for him and he obviously doesn't care enough about me to come and check on me. I'm not waiting for him any longer." I cautiously moved the covers aside and carefully climbed out of the bed.

The nurse could see there was no point in trying to stop me.

"At least let me get your prescription for pain medication and let me give you your discharge instructions," she said. "I'll be right back."

She came right back with the prescription and a piece of paper she said contained my discharge instructions. I was so annoyed that I did not bother to look at either of them. I was just hoping I could make it out to my car.

No one offered me a wheelchair so I walked slowly and carefully to the parking lot. I was weak and exhausted by the time I got to my car. I had been too sick to eat over the past two days and I knew this was why I had no energy. I opened the car door and got in with relief that I had made it this far. I started the car and slowly pulled out of the parking lot.

On my drive home, my mother's warnings went through my head over and over. How I wished I had listened to her. I was feeling guilty over how worried I knew she must be by now. She had no way to get around because I had the car. Besides, she refused to drive in Atlanta anyway. I told her I would be home on Saturday morning and here it was late Sunday afternoon. She must be out of her mind with worry. Our bond was so close that she probably felt every single pain I experienced over the last two days. I was feeling bad about that.

My drive home was slow. Thankfully, there were not a lot of cars out on the road. I was disturbed by the things I thought I saw out of my peripheral vision. I knew it had to do with the side effects of being on narcotics for the last two and-a-half days. Several times, I felt like pulling over on the side of the road. The only explanation I have for not ending up having an accident is that it was Sunday, and there were very few people out there. I must have been out of my mind to think I was capable of really driving home, but nobody had tried too hard to stop me.

Finally, I arrived home and pulled slowly into the driveway. Kendell saw me pull up and came running out of the house. He helped me walk inside. My mother met us at the door and looked at me with shock. She looked like she had seen a ghost. I could also see the fear in her eyes. Without a word she helped me up to my bedroom and helped me get into bed. She sent Kendell to the pharmacy to get my pain prescription filled.

For the next few days, I drifted in and out of sleep, afraid to move because it was so painful. The nausea and vomiting continued and I felt my temperature steadily rising. I could not eat. By Thursday, the pain medication was no longer working. The excruciating pain was back and I could not stand it. I moaned and cried pitifully. My mother was beside herself as she nursed me and tried to help me.

My mother called the doctor's office listed on the discharge paper. She called several times and received no return call after several hours. In desperation she called Dr. Snyder's office. She was able to reach him and she explained to him what was happening to me. He told her he would contact Dr. Langford and get back with her immediately.

When Dr. Snyder called my mother back, she was shocked to learn that Dr. Langford had not performed my UFE. Without my knowledge and consent, Dr. Langford had turned me over to one of his partners, Dr. Thomas Rowley and he had performed the procedure. Since Dr. Langford had told me I did not need a face-to-face consultation, I never saw either doctor and would not have known one from the other, even if I had seen Dr. Rowley at the hospital.

After learning that Dr. Rowley was the doctor that performed my UFE, Dr. Snyder began calling him instead of Dr. Langford. He called Dr. Rowley numerous times with no response. Realizing that my condition was worsening by the hour, Dr. Snyder admitted me to Butler Hospital. It was May 25th.

By the time I arrived at the hospital, my pain was out of control and I was nearly out of my mind. I was immediately given a strong dose of pain medication. I remember seeing Dr. Snyder and realizing that he had a very helpless look on his face when he saw me. I thought, why can't he help me? Or at least find the doctor that did this to me so he can help me. After all, you are the one that told me to go to Dr. Langford to have the UFE done. I trusted you Dr. Snyder. Finally, the pain shot began to work and I fell into a deep and welcome sleep.

I awakened and found myself in another hospital bed. My mother was sitting at the bedside watching me with so much worry on her face that I wanted to cry. However, before the tears could form, I felt the nausea rise in my throat and I started vomiting uncontrollably. I was aware that I felt feverish and hot. My mother touched my forehead as she was holding the emesis basin under my chin and I heard her gasp in alarm.

Once there was a pause in my vomiting, she rushed out of the room to get a nurse. I felt too sick and weak to do anything. I vaguely heard the nurses tell my mother to leave the room. They told me they needed to put a nasogatric tube through my nose down into my stomach to help stop my vomiting. I started fighting and screaming "No!" when they came toward me with the tube. It took two nurses to hold me down and one to put the tube up my nose and down my throat. Every movement of the tube caused more vomiting and I was screaming and pleading for them to stop. I felt like I was drowning fast, but I was unable to save myself. I was too weak to keep fighting and I suddenly found I could not fight anymore. They had given me another shot. I no longer cared what they did to me. My mind took flight into the world of oblivion, and I drifted in and out of consciousness for the rest of the day.

I came back to consciousness slowly but I immediately became aware of the pain again. I could feel the nasogastric tube still in my nose. I had several IVs and I was aware someone had inserted a catheter. When had that happened? I still could not move without causing waves of pain to course through my abdomen. I saw a nurse standing at my bedside. When I tried, I found that it was hard for me to speak.

The nurse gave me a pad to write on. I wrote that I wanted them to take the tube out of my nose. Please.

She looked at me and shook her head. "No, Kellee," she said, "we have to wait a while longer before we can take it out. We have to make sure your vomiting is under control." She injected something into my IV and I drifted off into one more deep and welcome sleep.

The next day, I awakened to find another nurse standing at my bedside. My voice was warbled but she understood that I wanted the tube out of my nose. I was surprised and relieved when she agreed to take it out. She pulled it out so fast that I felt water come up into my nose and I started gagging. The nurse quickly gave me an injection directly into my IV and I became light-headed once again. I started hallucinating, seeing objects that I knew were not there. They were coming at me from every direction and I felt that they were closing in on me. Soon, I fell into another deep unconscious sleep.

I woke up because I felt something being pressed up against my chest. I opened my eyes and saw a doctor leaning over me listening to my heart with a stethoscope. Seeing that I was awake she pulled the stethoscope out of her ears and said, "Kellee, I'm a cardiologist. I'm here because your doctors are concerned about the high level of infection in your body. They wanted me to make sure your heart has not been adversely affected by the infection. I'm concerned that you were not treated with antibiotics before your UFE."

I remembered then that I had always been pre-medicated with antibiotics for a simple teeth-cleaning. And the doctor had performed my UFE without giving me antibiotics? Didn't he know I was a previous heart patient? I became hysterical, my emotions spiraling out of control. I was frightened out of my mind. I was grateful when the nurse came in and injected a sedative into my IV and I fell asleep almost immediately.

I came to awareness realizing that somebody was trying to get me to swallow something. The gagging and impending vomiting had jerked me awake. I saw a nurse was standing over me attempting to force some contrast liquid into my mouth so they could get a CT scan of my abdomen. I fought it because I knew if I tried to swallow the liquid it would start the vomiting again. When I fought she threatened to put the nasogastric tube back in my nose. She threatened to give me an enema too. She was rapidly losing patience with me but I could not help it. Her attitude made be angry and I demanded to know where the doctor was that had done this to me. I demanded to know a lot of other things too. I was hysterical and out of control.

Before I could complete the list of demands I was so desperately trying to articulate, the nurse slid another needle into my IV, and my battle was over. As I drifted off into another drug-induced stupor, I remember thinking, why won't she let me stay conscious long enough so I can find out what's happening to me? Was there something they were hiding from me?

The next time I awakened, I lay quietly without moving. What day was it? I had lost track of time again. I was afraid to move because I did not want the nurse to come in and give me another injection that would put me under. I felt so weak. I had not eaten anything for approaching ten days. I wondered what caused me to vomit so much and I concluded that it had something to do with all the drugs they were pushing into my body through my IV. A feeling of desperation came over me and I wanted to get out of there. I needed to get to my mother so she could make me well again.

For the first time in several days, I felt I was thinking more clearly. I realized that I would have to control myself and quit acting hysterical if they were going to stop putting those powerful sedatives into my IV. If the nurses were convinced that I was better, just maybe the phantom doctor will appear and discharge me from the hospital. I desperately wanted to go home.

A nurse entered the room and I bravely put on a happy face in spite of the pain I still felt. "Will you please remove my IV so I can go home now?" I asked.

"Well, Kellee, has the doctor been in to see you today?" she asked. "The doctor will have to see you before you can be discharged."

"As a matter of fact, the doctor hasn't been in to see me yet," I said sarcastically. "I have yet to get up close and personal with the doctor that has caused me all this pain. If you don't pull this IV out of my arm, I'll do it myself," I threatened. "I'm going home."

Amazingly, the nurse believed me and proceeded to take the IV out of my arm. I must have put on a good front because I knew I did not have enough strength to push the IV pole to the other side of the room, much less attempt to stop her if she tried to sedate me again.

I called my mother and told her to send someone to pick me up and to tell Kendell I was coming home today. Later, I was released by a doctor who was not Dr. Snyder. He gave me a prescription for more narcotics to control my pain. Once again, Dr. Thomas Rowley could not be located. Obviously, he did not want to be located. I thought, is this what medicine had come to? Where doctors give their patients to other doctors without the patient's consent, only to be abandoned and left to suffer? An icy chill of fear was slithering down my spine and I got goose bumps all over my body.

I had not seen Dr. Snyder since the day I was admitted. Where was he? Maybe I should feel grateful. At least he stuck around long enough to get me admitted to the hospital.

On the ride home I solemnly reflected on my cardiologist in Ohio, and the kindness of the doctors and hospital staff during my hospitalization for my open heart surgery. They had been so attentive to my needs. When did it become acceptable to keep a patient drugged while the ball was dropped on her treatment and care? Did they actually believe that I was so delirious that I would not be able to notice the absence of the doctor who did this to me? I had never seen him. Did they think I did not realize that the drugs they kept injecting into my body to keep me quiet were actually causing my uncontrolled vomiting? All the time I was in the hospital, no one told me why my body was reacting this way other than to say I had an infection and that it was being treated with antibiotics.

I reasoned that there had to be more to this than just an infection. I had started feeling badly immediately after my UFE and it had gotten progressively worse. How can an infection warrant such agony? Am I cured now? I wondered. If only Dr. Rowley was available, maybe he could treat me, or at the very least, advise someone else on how to treat me. Why is this doctor avoiding his patient?

Once I arrived home, I went straight to bed because I was too weak to do anything else. It was May 28th. I did not want to be touched or even have movement near me for fear of arousing the horrible pain that was now a frequent and persistent visitor in my life. My mother was busy trying to keep me as comfortable as possible. I drifted in and out of sleep because every time I tried to turn, sharp knife-like pains would shoot through my abdomen and wake me up. In spite of this I felt hope because at least I was not stoned out of my mind on drugs.

What had happened to me was becoming a brutal reality. I watched my mother's concern and wondered how many times she wanted to say, "I warned you not to do this." But, she did not. I suppose she felt I was suffering enough. I was having plenty of occasions, of my own, to revisit her warnings each time the pain has burned like a white-heat throughout my abdomen.

Late that night I was awakened by the pouring down rain. It was coming down harder than I had ever seen. I lay very still and listened to the rain, afraid to move for fear of triggering more pain.

Suddenly, a strange sensation overwhelmed me. I thought, the angels are crying and that is why it is raining so hard. Could it be they were crying for what they knew lay ahead for me?

Chapter Four

The Road to Hell is Paved With Good Intentions

I was out of the hospital but the stalking pain had relentlessly followed me home. It had been ten days since my UFE. Over the next few days I began to fear that the pain would never go away. It seemed determined to continue to drill through my abdomen, mercilessly. Sometimes the pain was so severe, the only solution was to take another pain pill, even if it had only been two hours since the last one. The pain was unbearable and it was impossible for me to do anything when I was trapped in the throes of it.

I was angry for being forced to live in a drugged-out state, just to be able to tolerate my existence. I mourned the loss of all my excited plans for taking my real estate investment career to the next level. They were trapped somewhere in the foggy haze that overshadowed my mind on a daily basis. I could not garner any enthusiasm for starting my new adventure in the new millennium. What little energy I had was focused on coping with the unrelenting pain.

Railing against the doctors became pain-dominated pastime. How could they have lied to me so? They had to know that this was going to happen. Didn't they? Did they know that women experienced this kind of pain from UFEs? I wondered what woman, in her right mind, would ever agree to a procedure that would cause this type of hellish pain. Maybe that was why they did not tell me the truth about the after-effects of UFE. I would never have agreed to endure this torture.

One day, in my fogged-out state of mind, I thought of a dream I had just before leaving Naples. This same dream occurred three nights in a row. A voice kept saying to me, "Kellee, get your affairs in order." At the time I found the dream to be disturbing but, as time went by, it receded into the far recesses of my mind. Now, as I walked through my house like a zombie, the dream came back to my consciousness. I was frightened anew by the dream's implications, and I began to think that the dream had foretold what was happening to me now.

Did the dream mean that I was going to die? From fibroids? Ridiculous! Women do not die from fibroids! But, maybe in my case this was not true because something had definitely gone terribly wrong. My doctors had told me I would have some discomfort but that I would be able to go back to work in a couple of days. Here it was more than two weeks post-UFE and I was still experiencing the pain from hell. The pain had burrowed so deeply inside my abdomen that sometimes I wondered if death would be the only escape from its tormenting presence. Life was just not worth living if my fate was to endure this type of demonic pain.

I had trouble believing this was actually happening to me. It just did not seem real. I did not experience suffering anywhere close to this from my open heart surgery. The birth of Kendell had been a breeze compared to this. I kept hearing my mother's voice warning me not to have the UFE. If only I had listened to her! I wished so many times I could turn back the hands of time. Each time I realized there was no turning back, my spirits would plunge to the depths of despair. I wanted my life back the way it was before this hellish procedure but, somewhere deep inside me, I knew that that life was gone forever, and it frightened me.

Each day I kept hoping I would start feeling better but each day I awakened, the pain was still buried in my abdomen as though it had found a final resting place. I could not believe it had been fourteen days since my UFE. I was still having pain so sharp that it was impossible for me to exist without popping pain pills. The vomiting had stopped, and my mother encouraged me to eat yogurt and soft foods. She was worried about how weak and tired I was all the time. After all, I had been unable to eat hardly anything for two weeks. I tried to eat as much as my body would tolerate. I was determined to regain my strength and get through this painful interval.

It was slow going but each day I was able to eat a little more without the fear of nausea and vomiting. I started to get my strength back. At least I could stay out of bed for longer periods of time and I began to hope that the worst was over. I began to focus my will and my energy on gathering enough strength to drive my mother and Kendell to Ohio. Kendell was out of school for the summer and was excited about going to Ohio, as he always did, to spend the summer with his grandparents. He also looked forward to attending summer camp. We had long since stopped talking about going to King's Island. I wanted desperately to get Kendell to Ohio so I could come back home and get my health together. I knew I was in for the long haul, and I did not want him to witness any more than he already had.

We left for Ohio. It had been almost three weeks since my UFE. I put up a good front for my mother and Kendell with the support of the numerous pain pills I had to take to keep the pain at bay. I was able to drive as far as Cincinnati before I doubled over with pain. The pain got progressively worse even though I had been popping over-the-counter pain pills since I had left Atlanta. We checked into a hotel and all night I tossed and turned, rolling from side to side, trying to find relief. I finally fell asleep during the early hours of the morning. Before falling asleep, I prayed to God to just give me strength to drive the two hours I needed to make it to Columbus.

The next morning we started off for Columbus and we finally made it. My mother knew I was sick and insisted that I go to bed immediately. Exhausted and over-dosed from my pain pills, I fell into a deep sleep and slept until the next day. It was getting to the point that drug-induced sleep was my only escape from pain.

When I woke up I was determined that I would start trying to lead a normal life again. I decided to go visit my sister, Angie, who worked for Marshall Field's as a department manager. I was not going to stay in bed another day and I believed that staying in bed all day would make me worse. It was slow going, but I got myself dressed and drove with my mother over to my sister's store.

I walked into the store at a very slow pace and I saw that my mother was watching me out of the corner of her eye. I was not walking with my usual fast-clipped bouncy pace. We ran into some of the store employees we had known over the years, and I could tell by their expressions they were wondering what happened to me. I made it to Angie's office and was welcomed by a hug and a warm embrace. She and our mother exchanged pointed looks. I tried to put up a good act of feeling much better.

We walked around the store and I was enjoying looking at all the pretty things I liked. Suddenly, a sharp pain hit me so hard in my stomach that it knocked the wind out of me and I doubled over, unable to stand. Angie has always been a good person to have in a crisis. She did not miss a beat as she rushed me back to her office and my mother hurried along with us. Angie began stuffing my pain pills in my mouth as she pushed me gently into a chair. I was exhausted from trying to get my breath back. After a few minutes, my mother insisted that we go home.

Once back at the house she put me to bed immediately. As soon as I lay down the wretched vomiting started again. It continued for hours until it progressed into the dry heaves. The sound of my gagging tormented everyone in the house that night. I lay weakly in the bed with a waste basket clutched in my arms until I finally fell off to sleep.

I did not know what to do. Was this part of the healing process from my UFE? Maybe I was just one of those people who had a harder time than others. If I had really been critically ill they would not have let me out of the hospital. Would they?

I spent the next week doing absolutely nothing and I could only eat minimal amounts. It seemed like I was nauseous all the time. I struggled through the nausea because I knew I had to eat if I was going to get the strength to drive back to Atlanta. I decided I would make an appointment to see Dr. Snyder the minute I got home. I noticed I was spotting dark red blood and I wanted to know if this was happening because my fibroids were dying. My mother was having an absolute fit about me leaving. We were in the kitchen arguing about it one day.

"Kellee, I absolutely forbid you to leave this house," she said fuming with anger.

"I have to," I said. I had tried everything I could to persuade her that I had to leave. "I need to see Dr. Snyder so he can find out what's wrong with me."

She frowned at the mention of Dr. Snyder's name. He was definitely on her list of dislikes. "You're too weak to drive, Kellee," she said still upset. "There's no way you can drive to Atlanta in your condition. You can see a doctor here."

"That doesn't make sense," I said, not wanting to fight with her but still determined to get back to Atlanta. I dared not mention the spotting. That would really send her through the roof. "I need to go back to Dr. Snyder because he's the one that told me to have the UFE and he'll know more in terms of telling me what to do."

She shot me a sarcastic look that said it all.

"You've been masking your pain with those pain pills," she said, accusingly. "It's dangerous for you to be driving while taking all those pills."

"I have to go home," I said, as big tears slid down my cheeks.

I knew she would never understand but I had a strong sense of urgency to get back home and get my life up and running again. I was determined to do it even if I had to pop pain pills everyday. At least it was non-narcotic pain medication.

"Kellee, please be reasonable," she pleaded. "Who's going to be there to take care of you if you keep getting sick? You're too weak to drive and you're still not well."

"I've got to do it," I said quietly, wiping the tears from my face. I really was afraid to be alone but I knew I had to get back to Atlanta.

Back in Atlanta, I found myself, once again, in Dr. Snyder's office. I did not remember much about the drive home from Ohio. I kept the pain pills flowing and managed to arrive safely home nine hours later. As I sat on the exam table waiting for Dr. Snyder and Sheila to come in, I was hopeful that this visit would answer my questions and bring me relief from my pain. It was June 15th. It had been almost a month since my UFE.

I heard the door open. I turned and looked toward the door as Dr. Snyder and Sheila walked in. Dr. Snyder could not conceal the flash of shock that crossed his face as he stared at me in disbelief. I knew I looked bad and I had lost a lot of weight.

"Kellee," he said, with concern on his face and in his voice, "what's been going on?"

I repeated what I had already told him over the phone about what had been happening for the past month. I could not help crying as I talked about how horrible the pain and vomiting was.

I was still crying as I blurted, "Now I've been spotting dark red blood for the last several days and I don't know if this is normal after UFEs. Dr. Snyder, what's wrong with me? This is not what you described when you told me how I would feel after my UFE. You said I would experience some discomfort and be ready to go back to work in a couple of days. I haven't been able to do anything at all, much less work."

"Kellee, I know you're upset," he said, gently, trying to calm me down. "I'm going to have to examine you so I can answer your questions as to what's wrong."

I cried harder, bawling loudly. I could not bear the thought of Dr. Snyder touching me let alone examining me. I knew every touch would intensify the pain. "I don't think I could stand it," I said, sobbing.

"I have to," he said gently but firmly. "I'll be really careful with you."

And he was. Yet the pain still overcame my body and I clamped my teeth down hard on my balled up fist.

"It appears the fibroids have gotten larger," he said with surprise, as he bent over while examining me. I could tell he was distraught. He stood up straight, looked directly at me and exclaimed, "What has this man done to my patient?"

My body went cold with shock. The realization hit me that Dr. Snyder was clueless as to what had gone wrong with my body. Icy chills ran up and down my spine as it dawned on me that, if he didn't know what had gone wrong, he had no idea how to treat me.

Dr. Snyder was beside himself as he blurted, "And to think I never even received a thank you card for the referral!"

I sat up on my elbows and looked up at him with stunned disbelief. How could he possibly care about a thank you card from a doctor who lied to both of us about the UFE and abandoned me? What would the card say? Maybe something like, "Thank you for donating your so trusting patient's body to medical science. Because of you, I have gained a substantial amount of knowledge and experience on what not to do, next time. This will most certainly translate into an ever-growing source of increased revenue. Please feel free to refer any other unsuspecting patients into our welcoming hands. They will be greatly appreciated!"

I cried even harder as I lay back down. Through my tears, I sobbed, "What does Dr. Rowley say is wrong with me? Have you been able to talk with him about what's happening to me?"

Dr. Snyder was angrily pulling off his rubber gloves. He said, "I've made numerous attempts to contact Dr. Rowley. He still hasn't returned my calls."

There was an expression of frustration and helplessness on Dr. Snyder's face. Obviously, we both had been abandoned by Dr. Rowley, the phantom doctor who, tragically, had performed my UFE. His partner, Dr. Langford, the doctor who indifferently turned me over to him without my knowledge, authorization or consent, did not think enough of me or Dr. Snyder to return his phone calls, either. Dr. Langford was the doctor that Dr. Snyder referred me to, and he convinced me to have the UFE, but he obviously felt no responsibility to me as a patient.

I was at a loss for words and my eyes were sore from so much crying.

"Well," Dr. Snyder said, with finality, "we're going to have to do another ultrasound."

I was too terrified to object.

As I drove over to the other office building, I could hardly see for the tears in my eyes that rolled freely down my cheeks, unchecked. I called my mother to tell her what Dr. Snyder had said. I still could not believe it. She tried her best to offer words of comfort but it was no use. I was way beyond consoling.

Dr. Snyder's words kept playing in my mind, over and over, "What has this man done to my patient?" Even during the ultrasound, that is all I heard other than the whispering between Dr. Snyder and the technician as they pointed toward the screen. I could not get those words out of my mind, "What has this man done to my patient?"

The ultrasound confirmed that my fibroids had, indeed, grown bigger. Now they were equivalent in size to a 20-week pregnancy. My tears flowed even more.

As I walked out of the office, Dr. Snyder said, "Kellee, I understand your being upset. I'm so sorry but I just don't know what to do to help you. I'm going to keep trying to reach Dr. Rowley and I'll call you as soon as I make contact with him."

I could not say anything in response. I was too petrified. If Dr. Snyder did not know what to do, that meant everything he told me about UFE was a lie. And, if what he told me was a lie, then everything Dr. Langford told me was also a lie. The truth was both doctors had flat out lied to me. The proof of that was unmistakably connected with the horrible pain that continued to burrow deeper and deeper within my abdomen.

I do not know how I got home. I had not been mentally prepared to digest what I had learned at Dr. Snyder's office. All I could think was my condition was worse, the doctor who recommended me as the prime candidate for UFE knew nothing about the procedure, and both interventional radiologists had abandoned me and refused to respond to Dr. Snyder's calls for help. As I lay in bed that night, there was no escape from these haunting thoughts that continuously recycled through my mind. I finally fell into a fitful sleep.

The shrill ring of the phone, early the next morning, awakened me. Startled, I reached over and grabbed the receiver and found Dr. Snyder on the line.

"Good morning, Kellee," he said. "How are you?" Before I could answer, he hastily said, "I just wanted to call you and tell you that Dr. Rowley still hasn't returned my calls. If he doesn't call me today I'm going over to the hospital to find him. Here it is a month later and he still has not returned any of my calls and pages. I want you to know I have left him numerous messages." Dr. Snyder sounded really disgusted.

"Why won't he call you?" I asked, not really believing Dr. Snyder knew the answer. "We're having trouble finding him but he had no trouble finding me and sending me a bill for $7,500 for the UFE."

"What!" Dr. Snyder exclaimed. "$7,500 dollars! A hysterectomy only costs $5,000!"

"That's what his bill said," I sighed.

"I bet he'll respond to an attorney," Dr. Snyder blurted with obvious anger. "I'll call you sometime today, I promise."

True to his word, Dr. Snyder called me later that afternoon.

"Kellee," he said as he cleared his throat. I could tell he was nervous, and I gripped the phone tightly, preparing for the worse.

"I've finally talked with Dr. Rowley," he continued. He seemed to be struggling to find the right words. "I told him everything that was going on with you and the results of my examination yesterday. What Dr. Rowley said is that what is happening to your body is normal post-UFE." He paused before saying, "He said you could expect these symptoms for up to six months." Then silence. "Kellee," he finally blurted, "why don't you let me do a hysterectomy? That will alleviate your problems."

I was speechless. I could not believe what I had just heard and I felt pressure in my chest as though the wind had been knocked out of me. I was having difficulty breathing.

My voice was trembling as I said, "Six months? How is that possible? Dr. Langford said it was a simple 24-hour outpatient procedure. He said I would have some discomfort and be back to work in a couple of days! And that's what you said too! What do you mean, six months?" My voice was becoming loud and shrill.

"Six months. I know, Kellee," Dr. Snyder said quietly. "It's obvious we were lied to because this has turned out to be much more than a simple 24-hour outpatient procedure. So if you let me do a hysterectomy it will fix everything."

We were lied to? Didn't you know anything about UFEs? How could you be lied to? Six months? The thoughts were screaming through my mind. Was Dr. Snyder out of his mind recommending that I have a hysterectomy? The sole reason I agreed to have the UFE was to avoid having a hysterectomy. Had he not listened to me? Surely, I'd made it clear how important it was for me to keep my uterus? And, now he had the audacity to suggest a hysterectomy? After all I had suffered to save my uterus? My body felt absolutely incapable of enduring an examination let alone a major surgery!

"Dr. Snyder," I said, trying to control my anger, "I made it clear to you from the very beginning that I did not want a hysterectomy! The only reason I had the UFE was because you told me it would protect me from having to have a hysterectomy, ever! I haven't gone through all this suffering just to end up where I made it clear I didn't want to be in the first place! I wasn't even having problems with my fibroids!" Didn't he know I could not stand to be touched? Let alone be cut with a scalpel!

"But, Kellee," Dr. Snyder said, still trying to persuade me, "you might have to suffer uncomfortable symptoms for the next six months."

"Yes," I said heatedly, "How's that for a simple 24-hour outpatient procedure? But I'm not going to let you cut my uterus out of my body."

I lay in bed for three days. The shock of learning the truth about my so-called simple 24-hour-outpatient-procedure was more than I could stand. All the wind had been knocked out of my sails.

The first day all I could think about, over and over, was the conversation I had with Dr. Snyder. I could not believe it. I did not want to believe it.

The second day was the worst day.

I struggled to digest what had really happened to me. The horrible thought that my insides had been butchered kept torturing me. This thought reduced me to tears and a bundle of fear, fueled by not knowing exactly what I had to face over the next five months.

With cold shock, I realized I had been scandalously betrayed by these doctors. I could not fathom such treachery. Dr. Snyder had convinced me to have a procedure he obviously knew nothing about. How could he do this to me? What had been the point of the Depo Lupron shot? I should have listened to my mother. I trusted him and thought that he knew what he was talking about when in reality he knew nothing about UFEs. How could he turn me over to a doctor who would lie about UFE being a simple 24-hour outpatient procedure? I wasn't even having complications with my fibroids! How could he turn me over to a doctor that would give my body to his partner without my knowledge or authorization? How could he put me in the hands of doctors who would abandon me and not return his phone calls? What were their opinions of Dr. Snyder if they would not return his phone calls? Anyway, what kind of heartless doctors *were* they?

I was sick, very sick. And it was clear that the doctor who did this to me did not give a rat's ass about me. Maybe Dr. Langford had planned this all along. Maybe that's why he told me I did not need to come in for a face-to-face consultation. Maybe he already knew he was going to turn me over to Dr. Rowley and purposely neglected to tell me that. His secretary scheduled my UFE for that specific Friday so Dr. Langford would be the doctor that performed it. He knew I was going to Hillside Hospital just so I could have him perform the procedure. I found it hard to fathom the implications of this kind of deceit. I was sickened in mind, body, and spirit. Could it be the doctors did this to me for monetary reasons? Because I had health insurance that could pay for it? Because I am a woman? I could not tell which felt worse, the knife buried deeply in my back or the pain imbedded deeply in my stomach.

The third day I finally realized there was nothing I could do about what had happened to my body. I resolutely turned my thoughts to how I was going to make it through the next five months. I had already made it through one of the six months and in my mind I was counting the months down; one down, five to go.

I resolved that I would not be a cry-baby about this. It had happened and I had to deal with it. I felt so stupid for allowing myself to be tricked into something I knew nothing about. I believed in my heart that a huge part of my healing would require me to accept my fate and set aside my anger so I could get well. I would divert every ounce of energy for the purpose of making it through the next five months. By any means necessary. I had to if I was going to save my uterus. If I had to take my over-the-counter pain pills everyday, then so be it. Anything to avoid a hysterectomy.

It was a long five months.

Many days I was forced to go to bed because I could no longer tolerate the pain of standing on my feet. I spent many nights gripping the sides of a wastebasket due to uncontrollable vomiting. I fought depression daily. I tried to take walks to get exercise and to feel better but I didn't have the energy for it. Panting and out of breath, I would turn around and go back home. Eating was a chore and was only done for nutritional purposes. Anytime I put food in my mouth, I ran the risk of starting the miserable nausea and vomiting. I stayed close to home, never knowing when a horrible pain would strike me without warning. On numerous occasions, while driving, I had to pull off on the side of the road until the waves of pain passed. I was desperately counting the months until all this would be over.

Kendell came home at the end of the summer. I put on a brave front for him and used extra make-up so he could not detect how pale and drawn I had become. The ordeal over the summer had taken a huge toll on my body and I was tired deep in my soul. I was grateful that my family was in Ohio where they could not witness and detect my deterioration. However, my mother had never made peace with Dr. Rowley's prognosis. Every time she talked to me she tried to get me to see another doctor. But I could not stand the thought of more doctors in my life at this point. The betrayal had been too great. I wondered what it was about me that attracted people to me who would hurt and betray me? I could not stand the thought of a doctor touching my pain-filled abdomen. All I could think of was my mental count-down for my six-month sentence. Just two months to go and this will all be over.

The days seemed to be getting longer as the summer passed and the fall season arrived. The days only seemed longer because it was getting harder for me to struggle through them and keep Kendell in the dark about how bad I felt. I desperately looked for any sign of improvement no matter how small it was. If I made it through a day without nausea and vomiting, I took this as a sure sign of my being on the road to recovery, even if the next day the vomiting started again. At least I missed a day so that was something to feel positive about. I was determined to slay this UFE dragon and not end up having a hysterectomy.

There were times intense feelings of guilt and betrayal would overwhelm me. Guilt for having made a decision that resulted in this pain and suffering, and betrayal from doctors I trusted so much that I did not question their recommendation that I undergo a procedure I had never heard of. I felt that my body had been used for experimental purposes to benefit them, certainly not me.

I was still struggling with my abandonment issues concerning Dr. Rowley. I was angry with Dr. Snyder for ever recommending something that would bring so much torture and pain into my life. The thought that he suggested a hysterectomy still rankled with me. He seemed so knife-happy to cut out the reproductive organ I had so clearly said I wanted to keep. I was haunted by the fact that I had not been having any problems with my fibroids at the time the UFE was recommended. So why would these doctors recommend me for a procedure that had the potential of bringing me six months of this kind of persistent suffering? I would force these thoughts back with the mantra I had developed since I was told I would have to endure this nightmare for six months: One day at a time, Kellee.

Halloween dawned as a picture-perfect autumn day. It was absolutely beautiful and I started the day by going to the store to buy some candy for my trick-or-treaters. I did not feel well when I woke up that morning but I was determined I would not ruin this day for Kendell. I pushed myself through the morning believing my battle was just about over. After all, I was very close to the end of the six-month period Dr. Snyder had told me was normal post-UFE.

By that afternoon, I was experiencing a strange and abnormally sharp pain in my abdomen that was followed by nausea. I took pain medication and was careful to eat the small amounts I ate when I knew I had to battle this sickness. Still, the pain continued. I took more pain medication. The pain got increasingly worse so I took even more pain medication. I was desperate to calm the pain before Kendell got home and noticed my condition.

I could not fathom why I was going through a truly painful episode like this when I was so close to the end. As the pain intensified I realized, with panic, I was not going to be able to hide this from Kendell. Something was horribly wrong. When he came through the door, I found myself apologizing emphatically for my condition. The shock reflected on Kendell's face, in seeing me in such a terrible state, just about sent me over the edge. I knew I was beginning to panic and I struggled to regain control.

"Mom," he said, with fear reflected in his eyes, "we need to get you to the hospital." I feebly tried to resist but Kendell ran out of the house and got my neighbors from across the street. They came and rushed me to Butler Hospital's emergency room, that was not far from my house.

For an hour I lay, shivering, on a hospital gurney in the hallway. No one had bothered to give me a blanket. In pain, I cried and begged for someone to help me. I begged them to please call Dr. Snyder to come and help me. Anything but this pain. But I was completely ignored. It may be the hospital emergency room was very busy, but what about me? Weren't emergency rooms supposed to treat patients in need of emergency treatment? My pain was unbearable and I felt like I was dying. This thought bothered me and I decided I was not going to die in this hospital hallway. This hospital was just like all the doctors that had failed me and abandoned me. So, I left and went home.

Once at home I took more pain medication. I called my mother and I could tell she knew I was really sick. She kept asking me why I had left the hospital. I had no explanation other than I did not want to die in the hallway but I did not want to say that to her. I wanted to hear her voice one more time in case I did not wake up. I know these were morbid thoughts but I was not in my right mind. I called my best friend but I did not tell her how sick I actually was. I don't know why. I told Kendell how much I loved him and kissed him goodnight. As I fell asleep, I was not sure if I was going to wake up again but I took solace in the fact that at least I was at home and not in some cold hospital hallway lying on a gurney. I drifted off into a deep sleep.

At about one o'clock in the morning, I was jerked wildly awake. I was brought abruptly upright in the bed, my body trapped in the throes of projectile vomiting. At the same time, a cruel wrenching pain made its way through my abdomen in a snake-like motion. I screamed uncontrollably as I fell over on my side and tried to curl up in a ball. I continued to retch and I could not control the screams of pain in between the projectile vomiting. Frantically, I tried to slide my body off the bed but, as a sharp pain hit me, I fell to the floor. In panic and terror, I began to crawl across the floor on my hands and knees toward Kendell's room, still shouting his name as I made it into the hallway.

I saw Kendell bolt from his room and then come to an abrupt halt in front of me, gaping at me in shock as I groveled on the floor. Panicked at what he saw, he ran back into his room shouting that he was calling 911. He could hardly speak from the fear of what he had witnessed, but the 911 operator could hear my screams in the background. Although it seemed like forever, an ambulance arrived within minutes.

Kendell ran downstairs and let the paramedics in and they found me lying on the floor at the top of the spiral staircase. It was difficult for them to get the gurney up the staircase and even harder to maneuver it down with me on it. I managed to convey to them that I did not want to go to Butler Hospital and for them to please take me to another hospital. They assured me that they would.

As the paramedics wheeled me out of the house, I grabbed Kendell's hand and was shattered by the stark and raw fear I saw in my son's beautiful green eyes. He was trying to be brave but his fear was overtaking him. Somehow, between my screams of pain and vomiting, I managed to tell him to lock the door and turn on the alarm. I told him to keep the doors locked and to call his grandparents and tell them what had happened so they could come and get him. However, Kendell did not move and stood rooted to the spot as I was wheeled through the front door. He followed me out and then sat on the front steps and cried as he watched them put me into the ambulance. He was crying his heart out and I knew he was afraid he would never see me again, alive.

Once inside the ambulance I heard the doors slam shut. Through my pain and vomiting I was worried about my son being left alone. I was powerless to help him. I could not shake the terror that I was dying and that I was going to leave him alone and motherless. And all over fibroids! I thought once again; women do not die from fibroids! *But I knew I was dying.* It came clear to me in that instant that I had been dying for the past six months. I just had not known it until now.

As the ambulance sped through the city, sirens blaring, every turn and stop intensified the pain and projectile vomiting. Inside the ambulance, I spiraled swiftly into what felt like a surreal atmosphere. I felt like I was already entombed in a coffin because death was surely overtaking me. As I felt the strength draining from my body, I knew this was it. I could almost smell the Grim Reaper's fetid breath as I saw him bending toward my face so he could forcefully suck up my last breath, when I drew it. My terror knew no bounds.

Through my terror and hallucinations, I realized we had arrived at the hospital. The staff was waiting at the emergency room doors. As the paramedics quickly pushed me through the entrance, I was still vomiting uncontrollably. The hospital staff moved efficiently and competently to get me off the gurney and onto an emergency room hospital bed. They fired questions at me as they started an IV but I was barely coherent. I managed to tell them that Dr. Snyder was my doctor and to please call him. I saw a nurse run to the phone as they began to draw my blood. They must have given me a pain shot because, mercifully, the room began to recede as darkness descended over my body.

As pitch-black darkness finally overtook me, I was convinced that at the end of this six-month journey, I had been shoved into a one-way greased chute whose destination sign read, "Depths of Hell."

Chapter Five

It's Official You're Sterilized

I awakened to the sound of voices all around me. My eyes were closed but, behind my eyelids, I could see I was in a brightly lighted room. I cautiously opened my eyes protecting them from the glare I knew would be painful. As my eyes adjusted to the light I saw that several doctors surrounded my bed.

Noticing that I was awake, one of the doctors took my hand and leaned in close to me. He said, "Kellee, I'm Dr. Rivera. I'm sorry but we're going to have to operate immediately and take your uterus. We don't have any time to waste. We have to go in now."

I snatched my hand away. "Oh, no you're not taking my uterus!" I screamed. "I've just gone through six months of hell just to be able to keep my uterus!"

"Kellee," he said, "you don't understand what's at stake here. You have no choice."

"It's not going to happen!" I cried. I did not care what was at stake. They were not taking my uterus. Besides, how did I know if I could believe what these doctors were saying, anyway? Why should I trust them? I had been betrayed and lied to by three doctors and I was supposed to take their words as true?

Dr. Rivera turned and looked helplessly at the other doctors standing around my bed who looked helplessly back at him. One of the doctors was so frustrated that he turned and walked out of the room. At the doorway he turned and said, "We're going to have to send her home and let her die."

I had a flash of Kendell's beautiful green eyes, staring beseechingly at me. It was so vivid I gasped in surprise.

Dr. Rivera turned toward me, once again, with a determined look on his face. He looked sternly at me and said, "Kellee, you are dying. Time is running out for you. If you don't let us go in and operate you will be dead in an hour."

I started crying. "I'm not going to let you take my uterus," I said between my tears.

"You're not hearing me, Kellee," he said flatly. "You're going to die, and soon, if you don't let us go in and operate. If we can save your uterus, we will. There are a lot of things going on here that we don't have time to discuss with you. I need you to sign this consent form *now*."

My mind flashed back to Kendell. Was it fair to him for me to choose to die and leave him motherless? Was it worth trying to hold on to an organ that might cost me my life? I had betrayed my uterus' trust in me and I felt like I was agreeing to sign the death warrant of a close friend. Wiping my tears away, I reached for the clipboard with the consent form on it. I scratched my signature out on the line feeling as though the bottom had fallen out of my world. I had just lost the biggest fight of my life. One that I had fought so valiantly to win.

Almost before I scratched out the last letter of my name, the hospital orderlies rushed to push my bed toward the operating room. They were literally running down the hall as they dragged my bed along with them. The bed was moving so fast I could hear the wheels whirring with the wind that became entrapped within them. As I entered the operating room, I could feel the sense of urgency that gripped the doctors and nurses. They were moving swiftly to get me onto the operating table while barking orders on what to do next. I was aware of a doctor right above my head seated on a rolling stool. He had a gas mask in his hand.

"Kellee," he said, "I'm going to put this mask over your face and put you to sleep. Don't worry I'll take good care of you while you're asleep." The mask came down and covered my mouth and nose. The smell of anesthesia overwhelmed me.

Unexpectedly, it became the spring of 1981. I was sitting on the hill at Ohio Dominican College. In the distance, I saw a figure gently kiss the scar on my chest. Suddenly, the smell of anesthesia was replaced with the smell of Tuscany, and I was dropped instantly into an all-consuming blackness.

"Honey, this is Intensive Care, you can't stay long," I heard a voice saying. I struggled to clear the cob-webs from my head. My eyes felt crusty as I tried to pry them open. Once my eyes were open, I saw that Kendell was standing over my bed. He looked terrified.

"I love you Mommy," he said, in a choked voice.

I struggled to speak and managed to say hoarsely, "I love you more K, always remember that." I watched as the nurse escorted him out of the room.

I had no idea how long I had been here. I looked up at the IV pole and saw a bunch of bags hanging from it. What were all those bags doing hanging from the IV pole? There must be ten of them I thought with amazement. I tried to pull myself up out of the fog surrounding me but the effort was too great. I stopped struggling and let the blackness overtake me, once more.

The next time I awakened, I felt someone touching my body. I opened my eyes and saw that a sweet and kind nurse was sponging me off. I could not speak. I felt feverish and hot and my head felt fuzzy.

"Good morning, sleepy head," she whispered. "You've been a very very sick little lady. You've been running a very high fever."

It all came rushing back to me. Teary eyed, I asked, "Did they take my uterus?"

"Sweetie, I think we're going to have a new president, George W. Bush," she said to avoid answering my question. Before I could protest, I saw her push a syringe into my IV. After that, I drifted off into a restless sleep.

The next day I was moved out of Intensive Care onto the regular surgical floor. Dr. Rivera was waiting in the room for me when I arrived. I must have been somewhat better because I noticed how extremely handsome he was. Was he really that handsome or was I still under sedation?

With a pained look, Dr. Rivera said, "Kellee, I'm sorry but we had to perform a hysterectomy. Your case was critical and we had no choice."

I stared at him, unable to get any words out.

He continued explaining what had happened during surgery. "There was a mass involving your small bowel. When we opened you up we discovered that there were several loops of your bowel stuck to the top part of your uterus in the areas of the dying fibroids. When the surgeon tried to free up the small bowel, he saw that that part of your bowel had necrosed, in other words, died, and he had to cut that section out. The part that he cut out was also part of a large fecal mass. The dome of your uterus was plastered to the front of your abdomen. Your uterus was grossly enlarged and contained multiple dying fibroids. However, we were able to save your ovaries and fallopian tubes."

I ceased to listen to Dr. Rivera. All I heard was that my uterus was gone. Still, he droned on.

"We also had to perform an umbilical hernia repair," he said. "You developed an umbilical hernia from all your projectile vomiting." He stopped talking and looked questioningly at me.

I still could not speak.

"You wouldn't happen to know just what kind of instrument the doctor used that performed your UFE would you?" Dr. Rivera asked.

I looked at him and shook my head. Why was he asking me this? A red flag went up immediately. I said, "I don't even know him, much less what kind of instrument he used. You might ask Dr. Snyder, but, then again, he probably couldn't answer your question either. Where is Dr. Snyder?"

"Kellee," he said, looking pained again, "we called Dr. Snyder before you were taken into surgery and told him of your condition. He declined to come to the hospital."

He declined to come to the hospital? I was dying and he declined to come to the hospital? Another shot of reality flashed through me. Dr. Snyder had abandoned me, once again. He obviously wanted nothing to do with the mess he had helped to create. Something had gone terribly wrong in my body and, like Pontius Pilate, he washed his hands of me.

My mind went numb. I was having difficulty absorbing this. My uterus was gone. I had lost a close friend. I had suffered and endured the worse pain humanly possible for six months desperately trying to save my uterus. I escaped death by the skin of my teeth and the doctor who was responsible for setting this tragedy in motion, had declined to come to the hospital to treat me?

Unbidden, the tears began to copiously flow down my cheeks. I was crying in great wracking sobs, working myself up to hysteria. From somewhere, the nurse entered the room and gave me a shot. I was still crying when she walked out of the room.

Dr. Rivera was looking at me with genuine sorrow on his face. He patted my hand and said, "I guess you need time to digest all of this. I'll come back tomorrow and if you have any questions, I'll answer them for you." He turned and walked toward the door. At the door, he stopped and said, "Kellee, I'm so sorry we had to do a hysterectomy. I know how important it was for you to preserve your fertility, but we couldn't let you die."

Through my tears, I said, "Thank you for saving my life."

He gave me a long and penetrating look. Finally, he said, "I didn't save your life, Kellee. God did." He turned and walked out of the room.

I lay there, exhausted and spent. Eventually, the sedative took effect and I fell asleep. I did not wake up until two days later.

When I opened my eyes, the same sweet and kind nurse was in my room. This time she was applying lotion to my body.

"Good morning, sleepyhead," she said. "Do you feel better today?

"They took my uterus," I said, beginning to cry.

This time she said, "Sweetie, I think we're going to have a new President, Al Gore." She continued to apply the lotion gently to my body. Am I losing my mind, I wondered? What is she talking about?

The magnitude of what had happened to me was taking a firm hold in my mind. It was a good thing I was incapacitated because I really felt like a person with nothing to lose, and that could be dangerous. I'd lost my uterus through the incompetent and indifferent non-treatment of, not one, but three doctors. The emotion of what I felt was larger than the pain in my body. That was saying a lot because my whole body was one big bundle of pain. The only thing that kept the pain monster at bay was the pain shots regularly pushed into my IV.

I was no longer the same person I was prior to this experience. That person died on the operating table. I would never view anything the same again. If the doctors who did this to me were capable of this kind of callous treatment, the world was a much uglier place than I thought.

My grief for the loss of my uterus was slowly replaced with anger. It was evident to me what had happened. Dr. Snyder had referred my perfectly healthy body for a procedure I did not need and that he knew absolutely nothing about. How could he tell me I was the prime candidate when he knew nothing about UFEs? He sent me to Dr. Langford who parroted what he said but the deal had already been sealed with Dr. Snyder because I trusted him. I believed that, as a gynecologist, he was the expert and knew what he was talking about. That's why I would not listen to my mother. What did she know? She was not a doctor. Then, Dr. Langford turned my body over to Dr. Rowley, without my authorization, and he proceeded to butcher and maim me. All three doctors had abandoned me and left me to die.

These thoughts were too much for my hugely compromised and weakened body. I became extremely sick to my stomach just thinking about Dr. Snyder, Dr. Langford and, most of all, the doctor who maimed me, Dr. Rowley. I began to vomit. The nurses were scattering for emesis basins and trying to keep me from rupturing my still unhealed surgical incision. One was busy injecting a sedative into my IV. Through the pain caused by my vomiting, my thoughts were tormented. Did those doctors ever wonder what happened to me, or even care?

I still could not bring myself to look at my new incision. It represented something ugly and sinister. I touched the scar on my chest and reflected on how proud I was of it as though it were some kind of trophy. Whenever I faced hard times, I looked at that scar and knew things could have been so much worse in my life. It helped me to get through the rough spots. The scar on my abdomen represented something totally different, and I could not bear to look at it. It represented the epitome of betrayal, misplaced trust, deception, and abandonment. I wanted it off my body even at the expense of more pain because I knew I would never make peace with it. I felt as though I had been branded and tattooed by three heartless doctors who were determined to make sure I would never forget their betrayal. I would be forced to look at the scar that remained, everyday of my life.

Finally, the sedative came to my rescue and put me into a deep and welcome sleep.

The next time I opened my eyes I was astonished to find my room bedecked with flowers and balloons. I had no idea who they were from and I lacked the strength to get out of bed to read the cards. If it weren't for the balloons, I might think I was in the midst of a funeral parlor. How appropriate, I thought, an acknowledgment for the death of my uterus. It certainly fit my funereal state of mind. I had fallen into a deep depression and I made no effort to pull myself out. What was the point? No matter what I did I would never get my uterus back. My friend was gone forever.

I felt as though I had somehow betrayed my body through my blind trust and stupidity. I was always so careful to provide it with the proper nourishment and care. And in seemingly a blink of the eye, my good health was lost and I was suddenly engaged in a daily battle to win it back. And on this day, the score was not in my favor. The multiple surgeries and pain had drained my body of its strength. I had let my body down by so foolishly putting my trust in a doctor who would not even come to the hospital when I was on my deathbed. My guilt was enormous.

I accepted few phone calls while I was in the hospital. I cringed at the thought of having to put on a happy front when I talked to someone. I was just not up to the task. I knew I had a lot to be thankful for but it did not help. My neighbor had stepped in and taken impeccable care of my son until my mother arrived from Ohio. I was alive although I had come so close to death I could still feel the intense struggle within my body to mend itself from the onslaught of the multiple surgeries.

My mother had rushed to my bedside once she got to Atlanta. She looked completely drained when I saw her and I knew she had been frightened out of her mind for me. For once, she was at a loss for words to comfort me. The only thing she said was, "Baby, Mommy is here and I'm going to make you well again." She said this over and over during the days I was so sick that I was delirious and talked out of my head.

I remember thinking once when she said that, No Mommy, I don't think you can fix this one, ever. How could she give me back what was so senselessly taken from me? However, that did not stop her from trying. She was so happy when she took me home eight days after I was admitted to the hospital. I had weathered the storm and escaped from the clutches of death. That's all she cared about for now. Her baby girl was coming home and she would get busy making her well again.

My mother completely took over my care when I got home from the hospital. She waited on me hand and foot because I could do nothing for myself. I was still too weak and the huge incision on my abdomen hurt if I moved too much or too abruptly. She tried to be cheerful and make me think about my birthday that was only nine days away. I was grateful for her care and her kindness but there was no joy in my heart.

When my birthday arrived I found myself going through the motions for everyone else's sake. I was only thirty-seven but I felt old, very old. My body had gone through more at thirty-seven than someone who was one hundred and thirty-seven. That's how I felt. I had gone through six months of hell, gritting my teeth against the waves of pain, to end up losing my uterus after all. And to boot, I had been tossed indifferently on death's doorstep by three doctors who did not care enough about me to call and check on me during the six-month period. Dr. Snyder knew I was in bad shape the last time he saw me in June, yet he never called me one time to check on me.

All I could think about was the loss of my uterus; I would never be able to have children again. I knew I was single but I at least could have kept my options open, as long as I had the ability to have a child. I had not completely given up on that. I knew my biological clock was ticking but I still had time if I met the right person. Now I did not feel whole. What if I met the perfect person and he wanted to have children? And I was so ashamed of the ugly scar on my abdomen that I would not want anyone to see it. This UFE nightmare had robbed me of all my hopes and dreams. I missed being the woman that I was. It was snatched from me in the cruelest fashion possible and it was so senseless and unnecessary. These thoughts tormented me on a daily basis.

Two weeks after my birthday, I resolved to get out of the house and take a drive around the mountain. I had to make myself get out of the house and start acting as normal as possible. My mother had gone back to Ohio and I needed to get myself in gear. It was still difficult for me to get around and I had to go slowly as I moved around the house. I had been battling wild mood swings that I had been experiencing since I got home from the hospital. I would have abrupt hot flashes that made me feel so hot I could not stand it. Sometimes, I was consumed with a rage so potent that it would leave me feeling weak and shaky. I could not make peace with the injustice of what had happened to me at the hands of three negligent doctors.

It was these kinds of thoughts that pushed me out of the house that day and into my car. As I drove around the mountain I felt like a lost soul. I could not seem to clear the cob-webs out of my head and I had no concept of what to do to get myself started in the right direction. The exciting plans I had for the new millennium seemed to have flown the coup with my uterus. Actually, they had been gone long before then. I realized that a part of my life had been irretrievably lost the day I had my UFE. Nothing had been the same since then, especially my body which had gone steadily downhill. As I drove along, I was aware that I was engaging in a pity party but I could not help it. It was just not fair that this had happened to me.

I looked up and saw that I was driving past a new subdivision that had recently been built. When did that happen? I was in the real estate investment business and this had sprung up close to my neighborhood and I knew nothing about it. As I made a U-turn to go back to the subdivision, I was dismayed at how out of touch I was with things I used to have right under my fingertips. I pulled into the subdivision and took pleasure in looking at the beautiful homes. I was beginning to feel alive just doing something as simple as this. I was glad I took this drive.

Suddenly, I looked up and saw a house that had a powerful attraction for me. Well, I thought, I'll just go inside and take a look. Although I could hardly walk, I was determined to see the inside of this house. When I walked into the foyer I fell instantly in love with it as I realized this was my dream home. The house was extremely large for only two people, but in my state of mind, that did not matter to me. It did not matter that I had not worked for eight months. It did not matter that the house I was living in had not been sold or leased. It did not matter that I was short on cash.

What mattered was that I wanted to feel happy again and this house made me happy. I wanted this house. It would make all the ugliness I had experienced over the last eight months go away. I envisioned how it would look with the pretty furniture I would decorate it with. My spirits lifted as I thought about all the things I could do with this house. I felt alive for the first time in eight months and I sure as hell was not going to let this feeling go.

As soon as I got home, I called my realtor and got the ball rolling. I put my home up for lease and called my lender regarding financing and pulling money out of another property. I was beginning to feel like I was back in the game and it felt good. Maybe this was my start toward taking my real estate investment career to another level, as I had planned before my tragic UFE happened. I was able to put all the pieces together to get the house and I was pleased that I could move in it by Christmas. A new beginning was just what I needed. I desperately needed a new beginning in a new house with no bad memories.

Riding this wave of enthusiasm, Kendell and I went to Ohio for the holidays. I was still battling pain and sickness but the good days were becoming more frequent. That is, as it relates to my physical well-being. My mental and emotional states were a different matter altogether. I had become prone to emotional out-bursts for the least little thing. Kendell found me crying over green beans he refused to eat one day. It was that bad. My family treaded lightly not knowing what would set me off in the wrong direction. I was on a constant emotional roller-coaster and I was powerless to get off it. I'm amazed that everyone survived my mental fragility throughout the holidays.

My mother alluded to the fact that she needed to have a serious talk with me. I was avoiding it because I thought she was going to burst my bubble about the too big house I had bought for me and Kendell. I could just hear her telling me that I was being emotional about the house instead of being practical. I was in no mood to have my happy-house-pill taken away from me.

One day she cornered me and forced me to sit down and talk with her. There was no way to get out of it.

"Kellee," she asked, "just when do you plan to address what those doctors did to you?" She folded her arms across her chest and stared straight at me.

I was taken completely by surprise and was caught off guard.

"Address what?" I asked, scrambling around for some escape from this conversation.

"You know what I'm talking about," she said. "I'm talking about what those doctors did to you."

"Which one?" I asked.

"How about all of three of them," she said.

I had not thought about this at all. I squirmed in my seat as I struggled to confront the implications of what my mother was suggesting. Even though rage was a frequent visitor in my mind, I had not thought of retaliation. I was still too ill to find the strength mentally or physically to pursue this type of action.

"Now is not the time," I said, looking down at my hands to

avoid my mother's gaze. "I can't handle even thinking about what they did to me much less accept it enough to take some action against them. I just want to get well and move on with my life."

My mother did not push me and left it at that, apparently satisfied that she at least raised the subject with me.

Relieved that she had let it go, I continued my happy thoughts about my new house. I was looking forward to moving into my new home and thought it would be an escape from my painful memories. I could not wait to get away from all the baggage I carried in my old house. I kept thinking, a new start is just what I need to get going in the right direction. So, from Ohio, I closed on my new house in Atlanta, over the phone. When I returned to Atlanta, we moved into my new home on the first of January. Happy New Year! But I was sadly mistaken. What I thought was going to be a fresh start became a long extension of the nightmare, transferred to another location.

Right after moving into my new home, the pain started again. It was extremely sharp and centered around my navel and in my abdomen. I became terrified. What now? Why was I having these pains? Oh please God, not again.

Fortunately, I had a follow up appointment with the lead surgeon that had operated on me in November. The timing of this appointment was a blessing since I was now experiencing these peculiar pains. I was happy to go to his office and to be escorted to an examination room. I climbed upon the table and anxiously waited for him to come into the room.

When he walked in, he said, "Kellee Kendell?"

"Yes," I replied, "who are you?"

"Kellee, you don't remember me but I'm Dr. Thomas," he said as he walked toward me smiling warmly with his hand extended. He shook my hand. "I was the lead surgeon on your case the night you were brought into the hospital. You were already unconscious when I was called to the operating room at three o'clock in the morning."

"I'm sorry you were awakened in the middle of the night," I said, with a little smile playing at my lips.

He smiled back. "Kellee you were a very, very ill young lady," he said. "We didn't have a lot of time to work with. I'm so sorry we had to perform a hysterectomy. I know you didn't want that, but you look great now. How are you feeling?"

"As a matter of fact, I was relieved that I had this appointment today because I've been having very sharp pains in my navel and my abdomen," I said.

Dr. Thomas looked immediately concerned. "Kellee, during your surgery, we had to remove a segment of your bowel," he said. "It had to be resected, and put back together again with staples. The pain you are experiencing is, no doubt, coming from the scar tissue forming as a result of the bowel resection. That scar tissue is called adhesions. As for your navel, we had to repair an umbilical hernia that had formed as a result of all your numerous bouts with projectile vomiting."

I felt my mind drift off as he was talking because I did not want to hear this. It was still too emotionally painful for me. The seriousness of what had happened to me was hitting me like a ton of bricks. A bowel resection? An umbilical hernia repair? And last, but not least, a hysterectomy.

Dr. Thomas was saying, "Kellee, this scar tissue is very serious. It's nothing to play with because it's likely that it will increase. I need to refer you to a gastroenterologist."

Oh, no! my mind screamed. Not another doctor! Fearfully, I asked, "Will I need to have another surgery?" I could not stand the thought of one more doctor in my life. Besides, I was afraid to trust doctors.

"More than likely you will have to have another surgery," he said, with regret. "The scar tissue will have to be removed."

"I want to go home," I said as I quickly got down off the table. I wanted to get out of there in the worst way and run from what he was saying. I could not believe that he was suggesting another surgery at my follow up visit. I was still suffering from the last one.

"Kellee, would you like to follow up with Dr. Snyder?" he asked.

I turned and stared at him with disbelief. "What? The same Dr. Snyder that did not come to the Butler Hospital's emergency room while I lay shivering and in gut-wrenching pain on a gurney in the hallway? The same Dr. Snyder that declined, again, to come to the hospital the next day when he was called and told that I was on my deathbed? No thank you. Please don't forward my file to him. I'll be in touch." If Dr. Thomas would even suggest that I go back to see Dr. Snyder, I viewed him and anything he said with suspicion. He had to know what Dr. Snyder did to me. Did he condone that type of negligent practice? I realized with instant clarity that Dr. Thomas was not going to criticize the actions of Dr. Snyder, although he had to know that because of him and Drs. Langford and Rowley, I nearly died. So this is the conspiracy of silence among doctors that I had heard people talk about. I'll bet he wouldn't want to send *his* wife to Dr. Snyder.

Dr. Thomas seemed sorry he opened that up but the cat was out of the bag. I hurried from his office as fast as I could.

My drive home was long. I took the long route around the mountain to help to take the edge off of my latest health report. It seemed that this saga was never going to end. Seeing a gastroenterologist was the last thing I was going to do. Oh, please, I pleaded with my body, get well so I won't have to see any more doctors.

When I got home I opened the mailbox and received more devastating news. It was a letter from my health insurance carrier advising me that they were not going to pay my medical bills. It seems that they determined that my UFE was considered an experimental procedure and they did not pay for experimental procedures. Experimental? And, since my surgeries arose out of this experimental procedure, they would be considered as arising from a pre-existing condition and, therefore, not covered under my policy. I felt close to the point of collapse as my heart sank. My medical bills were so extreme that this would mean total financial ruin.

I just could not deal with it. I took refuge in sleep after fixing Kendell's dinner and I slept until the next morning.

Weary to the bone, I woke up feeling like a huge cloud was hanging over my head. It seemed that it was just no use. No matter how hard I tried, my life was determined to present me with daily challenges. I was sick to my soul of having to overcome one crisis after another. My mind struggled to deal with this new chapter created as a result of my UFE nightmare and I knew I had to do something.

All of a sudden, a slow anger began to permeate my whole body and every fiber of my being was consumed with a red-hot rage that was combustible. All the issues surrounding what these callous doctors had done to me came flooding to the surface with what seemed like gleeful madness. I had been avoiding confronting these demons, but now their flames were licking relentlessly at my consciousness. The powerfulness of my emotions made me feel ill all over again. I fought against the sickness that was trying to overwhelm my body and knock me down in defeat.

Ignoring the weakness that threatened to overcome me, I allowed the red-hot rage to provoke me into action. In that moment I decided that I was going to make every doctor that had done this to me accountable, or I would die trying. I shuffled through a stack of magazines and retrieved the one that I recalled having a list of Atlanta's top attorneys. I fingered down the list until I found one that handled medical malpractice. I was on fire. I found an attorney that sounded impressive and who appeared to be just what I needed. I made an appointment. After hanging up the phone, I telephoned the hospital and ordered my medical records, so I would be prepared on the day of my appointment.

I did not have long to wait. I walked into the attorney's office a week later with my medical records gripped tightly in my hands. I had to chuckle to myself when I met Jeff Matheson. He was the most self-absorbed person I had ever seen. Indisputably, he was tall and a very good looking man but he reeked with an unquestionable air of superiority. I could tell he enjoyed hearing himself speak but not as much as he enjoyed catching glimpses of himself in the mirror that was facing the conference table where we sat.

But these were minor infractions in light of the urgency of my mission. I needed an attorney and this one was listed as top-notch and that was good enough for me. He agreed to take my medical records and evaluate my case. Mission accomplished. I had no time to waste. I left his office feeling I had made a move in my life that would turn the tide in an upward spiral. I had faced my demons in spite of my fear. I was feeling proud of this one small positive move toward recovery. There was light at the end of the tunnel.

How could I know that the light at the end of the tunnel was actually a run-a-way demonic train headed straight for me?

Chapter Six

Far From Over

Each day, I became more intimately acquainted with depression. Before now depression was not something I had given a lot of thought. It was something that happened to other people and I had scoffed at people who allowed it to influence their lives. Just get over it! I would think if I heard about someone being depressed. But now I found myself in the same position—unable to get over it. I could not get over the senselessness of it all. Maybe if I had been sick from my fibroids I would feel better about it. But to be perfectly healthy and deceived into this hell of suffering, for nothing, was something I could not forgive nor forget. I was sure the doctors that did this to me would not be able to endure one hour of the pain I was forced to live with day in and day out. I went into a malignant rage every time I thought about how they were able to go on with their lives as though nothing happened while I was stuck with this hellish pain that resulted from their negligent acts.

Now I had plenty of compassion for people suffering with depression for I understood how you could not want to get out of the bed in the morning to face another day. I understood living with hopelessness that destroyed the very essence of your being. I understood the sick and frightened feeling that stayed in your gut and robbed you of any thought of joy. Yes, I had become intimately acquainted with depression

My mood swings added fuel to the fire and the hot flashes left me dripping with sweat and drained of energy. Many times I woke up in the middle of night so wet I would be shivering and cold. My bed would be soaked and I had to get out of the bed to change it. I slept in short spurts and could not seem to get a good night's sleep. This added to my depression and lack of energy and…the abdominal pain was increasing.

My mind would go back to my conversation with Dr. Thomas, who had said, "More than likely you will have to have another surgery. The scar tissue will have to be removed." The thought of another surgery alarmed me and I ate less and was careful of every morsel I put in my mouth. I kept thinking if I just took it easy on my stomach and intestines that would solve the problem and prevent me from having to have another surgery. I just had to be careful of what I ate and not put my gastrointestinal tract under any burden. These constant stresses caused the quality of my life to go steadily down hill. When my cousin, Malcolm, was killed in a car accident in February 2001, this added substantially to my already depressed state of mind.

I began to notice that I was becoming more forgetful and it seemed like the simplest things slipped my memory. This frustrated me because my mind had always been so razor-sharp that I worked circles around most of the people I worked with. Now I could not work at all. The simplest task might be destroyed by my incessant pain. The over-the-counter pain pills rendered me useless but I could not live without them. I don't know how Kendell made it through these difficult times. He was so patient with me and overlooked many of my infractions.

The months rolled slowly by. The pain kept coming. The bills kept coming. Then the financial difficulties started. This was no surprise as I was unable to work and had not worked for almost a year now. My savings were exhausted and I was getting behind in my bills. This terrified me. I knew it was a matter of time before my late payments would hit my credit report. I was distressed because my credit had to be impeccable if I was to be a successful real estate investor. My valued credit was the foundation of my livelihood and I had guarded it carefully for the past ten years. Now my very livelihood was threatened, and I was powerless to do anything about it. I could not bear what was happening to my credit and it was one more thing to be depressed about. I never thought I would come to this. The ongoing joke with my friends was that I would rather dance naked on a table than to get one over thirty on my credit report.

Each day, my life became more of a battle ground. Every day I had something depressing to deal with, be it pain, finances or sleep deprivation. There was no room in my life anymore for joy. So, when spring approached, I was not surprised to hear Kendell talking so soon about going to Ohio. I couldn't blame him for being in a hurry to get out of there. He needed a break from me. I needed a break from me but that was not possible. I could not escape the body that had been destroyed by the negligence of three doctors. Each time I thought about this I fought back the tears that welled up in my eyes. Sometimes I was successful at keeping the tears at bay and, sometimes, I would cry for hours.

When Kendell left for Ohio I felt so alone. I was happy for him but sad for me. As the summer passed I became paranoid about being alone in the house. I heard every little noise and I would lay awake at night listening tensely to the sounds inside and outside. My downward spiral and constant fear only made matters worse. I'm sure a lot of it had to do with my persistent insomnia for peaceful sleep was a thing of the past. One night after struggling to fall asleep, a car sped out of control and hit the back side of the mountain which was the side that faced my bedroom window. I was jolted awake and it frightened me badly. I was shaken up for days to follow.

The next weekend I was ripped out of my sleep by the sound

of firing muskets. The firing was coming from the local historic battlefield. It scared me out of my mind and I did not know what to think. The next day I learned that there was some kind of re-enactment of the civil war taking place on the battlefield.

It was the infamous straw that broke the camel's back and I could not take any more. I was tired of struggling to get well by myself and I could see I wasn't getting anywhere. It was no longer important to prove anything to anyone. I needed to be close to my family so they could help me. Admitting defeat, I packed up everything and hired a moving company to move my furniture into storage. I begrudgingly put my nine-month old house up for lease and went back to Ohio. Fortunately, the management company leased my house to a family that would take impeccable care of the property in my absence, and this took a heavy burden off my shoulders.

Back in Ohio, I was determined to concentrate on getting well but the relentless depression dogged my every footstep. It was September and I had been back for a little over a week. I cried the whole week sitting in front of TV watching nothing but CNN and the September 11 attacks. I could not shake my feeling of doom and gloom no matter what I did or how hard I tried and the mood of the country did not help my suffering. I thought if the pain would go away I could deal with almost anything else. But the pain was still with me and I was still popping pain pills just to make it through the day. In the back of my mind I would think about what Dr. Thomas said but I would not allow myself to dwell on it. I knew his words were grim but I was determined that not one more doctor was going to put his hands on me. Quite simply, I had ceased to trust doctors.

The Saturday after the September 11 attacks, my sister had a luncheon at her store and thought it would be a good idea for me to come to it and get out of the house. She thought I was watching way too much CNN. For the first time in months I fixed myself up and actually cared about how I looked. My mother was invited to go too so we left and I was determined to have a good time. All through the luncheon I was feeling proud of myself for getting out of the house. I had my mother and my sister by my side and that made me feel really good.

Suddenly, I was brought upright by a sharp pain that shot through my abdomen and cut my breath off. My mother heard my gasp of surprise and looked around and saw me doubled over. She had been through this before and knew exactly what to do. She got me out of there and back home. By the time I got home, the pain was so sharp and savage I could barely walk into the house. Once in the house, the wretched projectile vomiting started again. I was screaming in pain and terror. My mother dialed 911 and I was grateful to hear the sound of the sirens approaching within a few minutes. I continued to vomit uncontrollably. The paramedics moved fast and whisked me onto the gurney and into the ambulance. The ambulance doors slammed shut and I fell, mercifully, back into darkness.

The Emergency Room doors flew open as I was brought through the doors vomiting violently. My mother was running alongside the gurney giving the emergency room doctor an account of my medical history. Upon learning of my medical history in Atlanta, the doctor called the hospital where my surgeries had taken place and, miraculously, spoke to one of the surgeons that was part of my November 2000 surgical team. The Atlanta doctor remembered me well and was very descriptive of what had transpired in my case. He gave the emergency room doctor a wealth of information that he was not expecting to get.

There was compassion in the doctor's eyes as he attended me and ordered all the appropriate tests. I could tell he was very concerned about my condition in light of what he had learned from Atlanta. He reviewed the test results and they confirmed his suspicions. He introduced himself and gave me the bad news.

"Kellee, I'm Dr. Olson and I need to explain to you what's going on," he said. "The adhesions have blocked off a segment of your small bowel and your waste material cannot get through. It is poison for your body not to be able to eliminate its waste products. The adhesions need to be released and, quite frankly, your body is being extremely traumatized from your vomiting. I don't know how much more it can stand. We need to operate."

I started crying. I hated how helpless and weak I felt. I managed to say, "Please Dr. Olson, find another way. I can't stand the thought of another surgery. I can't bear the thought of another surgeon cutting me open again. I'm begging you not to do this to me. I'd rather die," I sobbed. I looked over at my mother for support. She looked distressed but she did not comment on what I said.

She turned to the Dr. Olson and said, "Kellee is very paranoid about having another surgery, doctor. Is it absolutely necessary?"

"My advice is to operate," he said. He thought for a moment then said, "I tell you what Kellee, I'll make a deal with you. I will take every appropriate measure to try and get your adhesions released over the next few days, but, if they do not work through your body, you will have to let me operate."

As they were wheeling me up to the hospital ward, I grabbed my mother's hand. "Mommy," I said, "promise me you won't let them operate while I'm asleep. I need you to promise me." She still wouldn't say anything to me. I looked over at my sister Angie who had rushed to the hospital to be at my side. "Angie," I pleaded, "help me out here. Promise me you won't let them operate on me."

My mother finally spoke up. "Kellee, I can't promise you that. If it means saving your life I'm giving my consent."

I was primed to protest but all of a sudden, whatever medication they gave me on arrival to the hospital, hit me full force. The pain and vomiting immediately dissipated and I felt myself spiraling into a deep sleep. As I spiraled down, the scent of Tuscany flooded my senses and made me forget all the suffering my body was forced to endure. I was in a deep sleep for almost two days.

I awakened and found that I could not move. I opened my eyes and saw that tubes and plugs where coming from everywhere. Even a nasogastric tube had been inserted while I was unconscious. I knew I really had to be out of it to not feel that torture. I hated nasogastric tubes with a passion and they would have had to fight me to get one down, if I was conscious. I remembered that it was September 15th when I came to the hospital. Tears flooded my eyes as I recalled the sharp searing-hot pain and the violent vomiting.

Dr. Olson entered the room. "Kellee, how are you?" he asked, pleasantly.

I found it hard to talk. "Please take the tube out," I said hoarsely.

"I'll take the tube out Kellee, but if you start vomiting again, I'll have to put it back in and operate," he warned.

I was amazed at the gentleness with which he pulled the tube out of my nose. I was so relieved to have it out.

"Kellee," he said, "we need to talk about the scar tissue that has formed in your small bowel that is causing this obstruction. It has to be removed. If not now, very soon. I have to be honest with you and tell you that your intestines are a mess and this will only happen again. My fear is that next time you won't be so lucky to survive another traumatic attack."

"If I have this scar tissue removed, will that be the end of my pain and surgeries?" I asked. "How will I know the scar tissue won't grow back?"

"We can't say that it won't grow back," he said. "It's more likely that it will, only in a different area. Unfortunately, in your case, surgery begets surgery."

"Well then," I said, "that determines my answer. No surgery. Why should I have surgery if it only means I'll have to have another surgery a few months later? It sounds like I'll just keep forming scar tissue. I'll take my chances with not having surgery." I looked at him teary-eyed and said, "All over fibroids."

"I know, Kellee," he said. "I heard the whole ugly story from the doctor in Atlanta. I'm so sorry this happened to you."

What did happen to me, I wondered. I still do not know. It seems every doctor involved with me knows the whole story but no one is telling me. I guess this is what happens when doctors close ranks. The conspiracy of silence rears its ugly head again. Who was protecting whom? And from what?

I was monitored closely for the next two days and then I was released from the hospital with a strict warning from Dr. Olson. He told me to be very conscious of any unusual sensations in my abdomen. I found that ironic because I could no longer identify what might be unusual sensations and what was normal. Normal was not something even remotely within my galaxy. His last warning was the hardest.

"Kellee, this will happen again," he said. "Next time you may not be as lucky to make it to the hospital in time."

Now what, I thought. Do I sit and wait for my next inevitable attack? I decided I would take every precaution to avoid another life-threatening event. With this thought in mind I, once again, monitored every bite of food I put in my mouth. I became extremely paranoid about food and any other upsetting event that occurred in my life. I had limited conversations with my friends and I seldom left the house. I did not like myself and what I had become. I did not want to talk to my friends because I felt all I had to talk about was my last hospitalization and how much I had deteriorated. I opted to not discuss anything at all. I would not play the victim role.

Soon after arriving home from the hospital, I received a certified letter from my attorney, Jeff Matheson, in Atlanta. I felt my heart plunge down to my toes as I read that he was not taking my case. My knees buckled. According to his explanation, his experts could not find evidence of medical malpractice in my case. I recalled the last conversation I had with him before he sent me this certified letter dropping his bombshell. I could hear his heavy southern accent as he said, "You wanted the blood supply cut off to your uterus, so they cut it off. They gave you what you asked for."

I was devastated. Whose side was he on? Obviously not mine. The gargantuan proportions of what I was up against hit me. It had apparently become acceptable to maim a patient and leave her to die. I might not be an attorney but something about what these doctors did to me stunk and I refused to believe they could get away with it. At least, not without a fight. If I did not pursue this to the very end, I might never know exactly what these three doctors did to me. The malignant rage was back and my anger began to eat me alive. The injustice of what had happened to me consumed my every thought and sleep became a luxury. Pain medicine, once again, became my constant companion. I was still suffering greatly and some narcissistic lawyer had the nerve to tell me I got what I asked for!

Malignant anger was behind the wheel of the car as I drove through the mountains in the middle of the night to meet with Joseph Fishman, another prominent medical malpractice attorney in Atlanta. I had done my homework on this one. I was told he was the best and that is what I needed if I was to slay the three dragons that so callously took my quality of life from me. I would be confident this time that I had my file in the hands of an attorney who really knew what he was doing. I was racing against the clock. There was a two-year statute of limitations on medical malpractice cases in Georgia and I was getting close to the cut-off. Mr. Matheson was thoughtless enough to sit on my case for ten months before telling me it was not worth pursuing. I guess I should thank him because he put the fire under me and made me determined to disregard my pain and make the trip to Atlanta in search of justice.

I was extremely weak and fragile and the predictions from Dr. Olson were constantly on my mind. I said a prayer and hit the road. I had a private talk with my body and asked it to please not fail me. I had work to do. I arrived in Atlanta in the early morning hours, completely exhausted. I caught some sleep and proceeded to the opposite end of town where I was to meet Mr. Fishman.

He was nothing like I expected. He was a handsome man with a very warm and a kind face. He was soft spoken. It was obvious that this man did not have to sell himself. His credentials spoke loud and clear for him. There was absolutely nothing that was abrasive or arrogant about him. He made it easy for me to tell my whole ugly story, and ugly it was.

At the conclusion of my story, he asked me what the prognosis was from my last surgeon. I hesitated only because it was so painful for me to say the words. I was reluctant to give life to Dr. Olson's predictions. Somehow, I stumbled through it.

Mr. Fishman looked directly into my eyes and said, "Kellee, you will have another attack."

I wanted to get up and run from the office. Now he had given Dr. Olson's predictions life and that was something I avoided at all costs. However, I did not run. I stayed and demonstrated that I was willing to fight every bit as hard as he would, if he took my case. I wanted him to see I was not a coward and that I would never give up on my pursuit for justice.

I left the office knowing I wanted Joseph Fishman to represent me and no one else. I had an incredible feeling about the integrity of this man. In the short time I spent with him, I knew he was a man of compassion and that he cared. I knew he was willing to fight for me if he found that I had a case. He told me he would get back with me after my file had been reviewed by his associate attorney.

Driving back from Atlanta, I had plenty of time to think about my meeting with Mr. Fishman and all the things we talked about. There was no escaping my grim thoughts. I was powerfully afraid of Dr. Olson's predictions of another gastrointestinal attack. Even so, the thought of another surgery frightened me more. From what he said, I might not be as lucky the next time. I was resigned to the fact that luck had definitely not been on my side, otherwise, I would not be in this mess in the first place. I had to be pretty unlucky to attract, not one, but three incompetent doctors into my life.

I had never questioned my mortality before. I was young and like most young people, death was something that was in a way distant future and not thought about at all. But the deterioration of my body had moved me much closer to the front of the line. I had come to grips with the fact that I might die at any moment. I did not share these thoughts with my family because I knew it would devastate them. But I had to think about Kendell. This was all the more reason I desperately wanted Joseph Fishman to take my case and fight for me. I could not die and leave here without doing everything in my power to secure Kendell's future. I cringed at the thought of leaving my family burdened with a ton of debt from astronomical medical bills and debt from my collapsing real estate investments. Time was not on my side if I had no control over when the next traumatic attack might strike.

As always, my mind went back to the thoughts that continued to torment me no matter how hard I tried to suppress them. My eyes filled with tears as I reflected on all the suffering I had endured. The part that got to me the most was that it was all so unnecessary. How could these doctors have recommended a UFE for a patient that had no symptoms? I was not suffering any pain or complications from my fibroids. I had taken the Depo Lupron shot. The magnitude of their combined incompetence never ceased to amaze and anger me. If I died, all three would be guilty of killing me but not one of them ran the risk of spending a day in prison. They would go on practicing medicine as though I never existed. I burned with the desire for them to be held accountable for what they did to me.

If I died, I wanted my tombstone to read, "All Over Fibroids." I knew Kendell and the rest of my family would never come to terms with what had happened to me. They would never get over it and I felt so much guilt thinking about how much pain my death would bring them. My suffering would be minimal compared to the pain they would endure as a result of losing me. They loved me so much.

All these thoughts played over and over in my mind as I drove back to Ohio. The fierce anger in the pit of my stomach grew and grew with each passing mile.

Once home in Ohio, I went straight to bed where I stayed for days. My depression was overwhelming. Sleeping was my only escape from the tormenting thoughts that overwhelmed my mind during my waking hours. I did not trust myself to be with anyone because, invariably, I would end up hurting somebody's feelings. My anger made me nasty and grouchy and I knew I was a terrible person to be around. I would explode in anger at the least provocation. It got so bad that my sister Angie cut off all communications with me. Her last words as she stormed out of the house were, "I'm not having anymore to do with you until you get some help and get on medication!"

That hurt. Still, I could not rid myself of the burning anger that made me impossible to live with. My family suffered a lot as a result of my ongoing demise. I would think, "What difference does it make? I'm going to die anyway and then they'll all be free of me." I had become a bitter and unpleasant person. I was hardly recognizable from the once upbeat and delightfully positive person my family and friends once knew.

As the days went on I could not shake the feeling of impending disaster. I knew my body was still affected by the adhesions because the pain was still there. And even if I agreed to the surgery where they would cut out the adhesions, more would grow in their place from that surgery requiring another surgery. Besides, I had no insurance to pay for a surgery because it had been canceled. There was no way out.

I was sad that my family's last memories of me would be so depressing. Memories of a sick and neurotic person. I only hoped that the memories of the woman I used to be would far overshadow the shrew I had become. I tried to discuss my morbid thoughts with my mother but she refused to listen to such talk. Her refusal frustrated me because, for the sake of Kendell, there were so many things she needed to understand. Why wouldn't she listen to me? She had heard the same dire predictions from Dr. Olson that I had. My mother was usually a very reasonable person but this time she had the blinders firmly in place. I felt she was in complete denial of my true circumstances but her denial would not make them go away.

It was three weeks since my meeting with Mr. Fishman and I had not heard from him. I was anxious and nervous about what might be going on. With apprehension, I called his office fully expecting to hear bad news. Instead, he sounded pleased to hear from me and advised me that I would be getting a call from his office within the next couple of days.

Two days later, my mother called me to the phone whispering that it was Mr. Fishman's office on the line.

"Hello?" I said.

"Hello, Kellee, my name is Phyllis Marks," a voice said. "I'm the nurse-attorney that has been evaluating your medical records over the past few weeks." She had a very pleasant voice and for some reason, it had an immediate calming affect on me. I could not remember the last time I felt this kind of calmness.

She said, "According to my initial evaluation of your medical records, in conjunction with my medical literature research, we believe we should take the next step with your case and send it to experts. In your case, we need two different experts. We need an Ob/Gyn and an interventional radiologist. The reason for two experts is that we need to have one expert review Dr. Snyder's conduct and another expert to review Dr. Langford and Dr. Rowley's conduct. We're encouraged by what we have found in the medical literature."

As I listened to her, my feelings about her were incredible. I was taken in by her demeanor, and every word she said to me was like salve to my soul. I listened as she went to great lengths to explain everything so that I would understand what was going on with my case. I knew I was not going to remember everything she said but the high points stayed in my mind.

"Do you think the experts will find negligence?" I asked hesitantly. I remembered that Jeff Matheson's experts had not.

Her response was swift and sure. "From what I'm seeing in the medical literature, Kellee, I don't see how they could not find negligence," she said. "According to my research, you should never have had a UFE in the first place. My research indicates that women who are interested in preserving their fertility are not appropriate candidates for this procedure. Even more important, you were not having symptoms from your fibroids. There is a serious question that the follow-up care of Dr. Langford and Dr. Rowley was within the standard of care accepted in the medical community. There is also a question of the appropriateness of Dr. Langford turning you over to Dr. Rowley without your authorization and consent. These are all questions that we will have answered once we send your file to our experts."

As I listened to Ms. Marks, I could hear the compassion in her voice for all I had endured. It was clear to me that this woman was fully involved in my case and would do all that was necessary to see that it was prepared effectively and efficiently for the experts. She knew everything about my hospitalizations and about every doctor that had been involved in my care. I was impressed. It was as though she knew everything about me even beyond what was in my medical records. She had the innate ability to win my confidence just by her style of delivery and the genuine warmth she conveyed throughout the conversation. I remember thinking that this is a woman that meets no strangers because I was instantly comfortable with her. It did not surprise me that Mr. Fishman was in association with such a person. They complimented each other.

By the time I hung up the phone, I was in an unbelievable

state of relief. I was basking in Ms. Marks' confidence and strength. She was like water to my parched and dying soul. Intuitively, I knew that she would never be accused of being a fence straddler regardless of other people's opinions. The attributes I recognized in her were once attributes I possessed before I became so beaten down from my illness. Having your quality of life so senselessly stripped from you can do that to you.

I felt good that day after talking to Ms. Marks, and I had a few days of hope that the tide in my life was really changing. However, that was not to last for long.

That late February night was unusually cold and dark. Its icy and freezing chill was fitting for what was about to happen to me. In the early morning hours, I was struck, once again, with horrendous pain that induced uncontrollable and projectile vomiting. This was it. The moment we had all been dreading but that was predicted to happen. I knew I was going to die. No one in the family had been willing to accept this possibility but me. I knew this moment was coming. I knew I would not be able to endure the horrendous pain that was now attacking my body, for much longer.

What an awful way to die, I thought. Will I strangle to death on my vomit or will my body be merciful and just shut down and provide me with a quick ending? At least I deserved to die quickly after suffering non-stop for almost two years. I felt sorry for my family that would be forced to give their last goodbyes to Kendell's mother, Marlene's daughter, Angie's only sister, and Darin's aunt. They have been my world forever, but they all refused to listen or understand the need to prepare for this day. My only release from this pain from the pit of hell was death.

Everyone in the house was aroused and gripped by my screams of terror caused by the escalating pain and vomiting. As my mother frantically tried to get me ready to go to the hospital, I kept collapsing on the floor. She had already dialed 911 and was kneeling on the floor next to me trying to wipe me down with a cold cloth. Kendell refused to come out of his room and was talking to me through the closed bedroom door. He was too terrified to see me in this condition.

My soul had accepted the inevitable but greatly feared the unknown. I just wanted to get it over with. This time the fight had gone out of me, my body was tired and worn out, and I no longer had the strength to go through one more traumatic episode. But not my mother. I knew she was fighting for me and refused to accept that this was the end for me. She had become an expert at orchestrating all the moves to get me rapidly in the ambulance once the paramedics arrived. The paramedics were familiar with my circumstances from all the other times they had come to this house. Like my mother, they knew time was of the essence.

The ambulance doors slammed shut, once again, and as we sped through the darkened streets, my thoughts flew to my case in Atlanta. The pain that was attacking my body was relentless and cruel. Through the murky grogginess that was overtaking my mind, I desperately hoped that I would get one more chance to speak to Ms. Marks. I had no confidence that this would happen. Desperately, my mind screamed in silence as though she could hear me…Please proceed without me!

Chapter Seven

Angel on Peachtree Street

The darkness of the soul can be so black that no amount of light can penetrate it. Fear can grip your heart so tightly that you can feel the breath of life being slowly squeezed from your body. Pain can reach such proportions that the torture of it propels you to plead with God to be merciful and grant you death. I had arrived at that point in my life.

It was déjà vu. Everything that happened when I was forced to have my emergency surgeries in November 2000 was now happening in February 2002. The pain attacking my body was so vicious I was convinced it was devised by demons that lived in the pit of a fiery hell. The vomit that spewed forth from my mouth came in vile green torrents. If someone had thought to video record it, they would have been paid handsomely by Hollywood for its use in the next exorcist movie. Special effects would have been unnecessary for this scene.

IVs were attached, once again, to my body, and I had been told they were going to have to insert the wretched nasogastric tube to control my vomiting. Mercifully, Dr. Olson had come quickly to my bedside and ordered immediate sedation. When I came to, he was standing over my bed gently rubbing my forehead.

Tears filled my eyes as I looked up at him with guilt.

"Are you mad at me?" I asked.

"Why would I be mad at you Kellee?" he asked.

"Because you warned me in September, if I didn't allow you to operate, this would happen," I sobbed.

"Kellee, you were so scared, and you had already been through so much," he said. "I don't blame you for not wanting surgery that might beget another surgery."

He continued to rub my forehead as I shed silent tears.

"I'm going to have to get a CT scan to confirm my suspicions," he said, knowing I would hate it.

I was too terrified to ask what his suspicions were. I did not want to know. My heart sank as I thought about the contrast medium I would have to drink in order for the CT scan to be performed. I knew if I tried to swallow it, I would start vomiting again, and that would make the insertion of the nasogastric tube imperative. As it turned out, Dr. Olson had to have me sedated for the test to be performed.

The next morning I woke up and discovered that the nasogastric tube had been inserted. My mother was at my bedside. She was waiting for Dr. Olson to come to the hospital to tell us the results of the CT scan.

When Dr. Olson arrived he got right to the point.

"Kellee," he said, "it's just as I suspected, you have a bowel obstruction, and we have to go in and operate."

My worst fears had come to pass. I turned my gaze down to my tightly clasped hands. When I raised my head, I looked straight into Dr. Olson's eyes and said, "If you get inside and you find that I'll have to live the rest of my life with a bag attached to my stomach, let me die." I meant it. I knew I had to have this surgery in order to live, but I would rather die than live with a colostomy.

Dr. Olson looked at me with compassion but did not respond. His touch on my forehead was soft before he turned and walked out of the room.

In my heart I did not believe I would survive this surgery anyway. The pain I'd suffered over the last five months had to mean things were really bad inside me. I had not forgotten Dr. Olson's grim predictions back in September. If his predictions were that bad then, five months later, if I was still having pain, things just had to be worse. But in the slim chance that I did make it, I wanted to make my requests clear. I looked up at my mother.

"I want you to call Phyllis Marks and tell her what happened," I said. "Tell her to please continue to fight my case even if I die."

My mother's face was full of love as she looked down at my face and into my tear-filled eyes. "I'll call Ms. Marks," was all she would say as she stroked my hair.

Still in denial I thought, but I understood. My mother would never concede that death was a possibility for me.

I settled back in the bed, resigned to my fate. I believed with all my heart that Ms. Marks would understand how I felt even if I died. I believed that she would not let death silence me and leave my story untold. I was comforted as I realized that she was my guardian angel sent by God to pick up my blood stained banner and carry it to victory for me, if necessary. Whether I was alive or dead, she was the chosen one to replace the strength I no longer had. God knew exactly what He was doing when He sent her into my life.

My sister arrived at the hospital and she and my mother stayed with me until I was taken into surgery. Kendell did not come because he could not face seeing me like this and, quite frankly, I was glad he was not here. He had been traumatized enough and I wanted to spare him this latest pain. I felt I had somehow failed him even if it had not been intentional. For almost two years he witnessed his wonderfully vibrant mother being steadily reduced to a mere shadow of what he remembered her to be for all of his life.

As I was being wheeled into the operating room, Angie and

my mother kissed me on my forehead and reiterated their love for me. I told them I loved them too. I looked longingly at them as I drank in every aspect of their precious faces. I wanted to carry a vivid memory of them into surgery in case I never saw them again.

In the operating room the mask was placed over my face. This time the anesthesia was not replaced with the smell of Tuscany. It was just as well because that scent represented a different form of betrayal and trust. It would not be befitting for that to be my last memory of my life here on earth. As the blackness began to overtake me, my mind was transported to Jamaica where I saw myself riding a jet ski just before sunset. In the next instant I was on the back of my friend's motorcycle riding up in the mountains, headed towards Ricks Café to conclude the evening cliff diving.

Jamaica....

I woke up in the recovery room. It slowly dawned on me that I was still alive. I was barely conscious. I couldn't feel anything but I was aware that tubes, IVs and machines, were attached to my body. I heard the sound of voices just outside my room. Although my vision was blurred, my hearing was oddly razor-sharp.

"What in the world happened to her?" a voice asked that I did not recognize.

"It was due to a botched up mess in Atlanta," the second voice replied. It was Dr. Olson.

Botched up mess? He never told me that although I had asked many times what happened to me. Before I could think about it anymore, I slipped back into darkness.

I was released from the hospital a week after my admission. I went through the same hell I experienced with my first surgeries except my recovery was more difficult. I was beaten down and my mental state was rapidly deteriorating. I felt such a rage within my body that at times it was beyond tolerance and I would explode with anger at the least provocation. I did not know whether it was from a chemical imbalance in my body that precipitated constant hot flashes, or whether the trauma of my second surgeries was just too much for me to bear.

At home, my recovery was slow and painful. I felt myself falling into a deeper and darker depression. I had been this way in the hospital too. Dr. Olson had talked at length with me about what had occurred with my bowel obstruction this time.

"It's a good thing we got in there and operated, Kellee," he had said. "When we opened you up, you had a large amount of thin watery fluid in your abdominal cavity and we suctioned this out. Your abdomen was full of adhesions. Some of your adhesions had wrapped tightly around a segment of your intestines like a rubber band. They were causing a narrowing of the bowel that caused it to become blocked. Your bowel was literally being strangled. We had to cut out that blocked portion of your bowel and then reconnect you bowel back together with surgical staples. We cut through the remaining adhesions and removed them. We also found that you had developed another umbilical hernia, caused by your projectile vomiting, and we had to repair it before closing you back up."

"Has my nightmare ended?" I had asked Dr. Olson.

"Kellee, you should expect the worse and hope for the best," he had responded, sadly.

Expect the worse, hope for the best. I guess that said it all. It sounded like a life sentence of torture and it produced in me fear, worry, and anticipation of another such attack. After all, Dr. Olson had said before, in my case, surgery begets surgery. Abdominal adhesions would form each time I had surgery with the potential of causing another bowel blockage.

With this prognosis I could not feel good about anything. I was afraid to eat, afraid to sleep. I knew I had to accept the hand I was dealt but I found this so hard to do. It was hard to accept that my life had become this tragic because of a UFE I did not even need.

My thoughts became suicidal. I began to ask myself if life was worth living with this kind of sentence hanging over my head. Before this, I viewed suicide as a selfish and cowardly act. Now it became more attractive as I endured the endless pain, depression, and sleep deprivation. My downward spiral was escalating. It seemed as though my emotional and physical scars had become conjoined into one huge accumulation of daily torture.

Even though I thought of suicide I knew in my heart I would never do it. But I did develop more compassion for people who chose this as an option. I loved Kendell and my family too much to saddle them with the emotional burden of my suicide. Besides, my religious beliefs were ingrained too deeply. God would never forgive me for such an act. I was trapped with this life of pain and suffering. I wondered what in the world I had sowed to be reaping on such a huge scale. I had become a pain-ridden basket case.

I knew I had to do something, so when Dr. Olson recommended that I start taking Paxil, I did not leave his office bucking and kicking. I had previously believed that antidepressants were for weak people unable to take control of their lives. Well, I had joined the crowd and it was teaching me a definite lesson in humility.

Through it all, I never gave up on my determination to pursue retribution for my needless pain and suffering, even if it took the rest of my life. So when the call came from Ms. Marks, it was like a ray of sunshine into my dark and painful life.

"Hello, Kellee?" she said, "This is Phyllis Marks calling from Joseph Fishman's office. How are you doing today?"

"I'm feeling a lot better," I replied delighted to hear from her.

"I was sorry to hear that you had to be readmitted but I'm glad things turned out okay for you." She paused then said, "We've heard from two of the experts and I have some good news for you."

"Really?" I said. "What did they say?" I could detect the restrained excitement in her voice.

"As I told you before, we submitted your file for review to two different types of experts," she said. "Two interventional radiologists and two Ob/Gyns. We've gotten a response from one of each. I'll start with the interventional radiologist first."

I could hear her shuffling papers in the background as I nervously waited for her to continue.

"Dr. Lawrence Kirby is the interventional radiologist that reviewed your file. He said that it is the responsibility of the interventional radiologist to tell you that you may not preserve your fertility if you choose to have a UFE. Not only that, you should be told that you may end up losing your uterus. It's part of the risk of this procedure. Although he believes that your risk of hysterectomy is higher with a myomectomy, which is where they surgically remove the fibroids from your uterus, you have to be informed of all the risks associated with UFE. That's point number one.

"The second point is that, in his opinion, it was the responsibility of Dr. Rowley to tell you the risks of the procedure. He believed that Dr. Snyder could tell you about UFE as an alternative procedure, but since he did not perform it, he felt he did not know enough to give informed consent. He didn't feel that it was really Dr. Snyder's responsibility to go over the procedure with you. Are you following me so far?"

"Yes, I am," I responded, and she continued.

"The third point is that he didn't believe the Depo Lupron shot had a chance to do anything because of the very short time it was in your system prior to your UFE. He thought that for it to have any effect in two to three days is extremely unlikely although he did not think there was a consensus among physicians about how to handle Lupron. However, his opinion is that most would agree that the very short interval you were on it would have very little or no impact on the technical performance of the procedure. I know this is a lot for you to digest so if you have any questions while I'm talking please interrupt me and I'll try to answer them for you. Okay?"

"That's fine. Right now I don't have any questions." I could barely contain my excitement and I was anxious to hear the rest.

"The fourth point is that Dr. Kirby thought there is a strong case against Dr. Rowley for not taking responsible care of someone that he performed a procedure on. He did say he had no idea if there was some totally unusual circumstance that interfered with his ability to give you proper follow up care, although he found it pretty hard to find a reasonable defense to this, based on your records."

"They didn't give me follow up care, they abandoned me and left me to die," I could not help but interject. I felt very strongly on this point and it still rankled with me.

"I understand why you feel that way Kellee," Ms. Marks said and I could hear the compassion in her voice. She continued.

"The fifth point we discussed was the issue of the coils. Dr. Kirby explained that, when used by doctors, the coils are put in at the end of the UFE procedure. The purpose for the use of coils is to seal the uterine artery closed after sending the polyvinyl alcohol particles to cut off all the blood supply to the fibroids. He said that most doctors quit using the coils about a year or two ago, at least. It seemed that doctors learned that the pain after the procedure was more severe with the use of coils. When you go to the point of completely blocking the flow of blood to both uterine arteries, he thought most doctors would agree you increase the risk of rendering the uterus more ischemic. Ischemia simply means you are cutting the blood supply off to an organ. When that happens, necrosis, or in other words, death of that organ can occur.

"The sixth point is the issue of the prophylactic use of antibiotics. Dr. Kirby said that when a UFE is done, not everyone gets antibiotics. He does not know of anyone who keeps patients on antibiotics beyond a single dose at the time of the UFE."

"Well," I said, "it sounds like you went over a lot with him. It's a lot to comprehend."

"We try to cover the important points so we can get a better idea of what we are dealing with. I know you're not going to remember everything but that's not your responsibility. Anytime you have any questions about anything, you just pick up the phone and call me and I'll try to answer them." Ms. Marks said.

"The seventh and final point is the issue of whether it is common to have pain for six months after this procedure. Dr. Kirby said, if Dr. Rowley stated it was not uncommon to have pain or bleeding for six months, that is downright wrong. He said pain and bleeding for six months is not a normal finding. It means there is a failure in the procedure. You can have spotting periodically for the first month or two, but if bleeding persists after that, most doctors would follow up on it. It is not common to have pain for six months. You have pain for maybe a week after the procedure, maybe some soreness for a couple of weeks, but like any surgery, you are past the stage of healing and into recovery by this time. He believes that once Dr. Rowley was contacted by Dr. Snyder, he should have made an effort to follow up. In your case, Dr. Rowley should have taken further action with imaging to make sure the fibroids were dead or just what is going on. But Dr. Rowley did nothing."

It was difficult for me to hear this. I was happy to finally be getting some information about what happened in my case, but it cut me to the quick to hear that what Dr. Rowley had told Dr. Snyder about the six-month period, was absolutely wrong. I thought about how I had struggled so hard to make it through those six months because I thought I had not choice. I felt my anger flaring up again.

"In a nutshell," Ms. Marks was saying, "Dr. Kirby believes a lot of things went wrong with your care in terms of Dr. Langford and Dr. Rowley. He thought the follow up care was negligent. He said Dr. Rowley should have been following up by phone when you were not doing well. He does not believe you should have been home and miserable for three days and then readmitted by the Ob/Gyn because Dr. Rowley was no where to be found. He said it's hard to say whether your outcome would have been different but it certainly seemed to him that your whole course became long and protracted, and probably with a little more diligence, up front, they might have been able to intercede on that cycle of pain and inflammation, and maybe even altered your course. His gut instinct was that if Dr. Rowley had been more on the ball, none of this would have happened. He thought the whole thing went on and on and finally the inflammation was so severe that your bowel got stuck to your uterus.

"He felt they should have gotten an MRI to see what was going on. He would have brought you back to the hospital, given you hydration and antibiotics and seen you through the first episode. Then you might have gone home and come back three weeks later with the cramps and pain. Then he would have gotten another MRI and made sure everything was okay. He felt you were being left with a situation that was not likely to have gotten better all by itself, and Dr. Rowley needed to be on top of things. He did say what he was doing was Monday morning quarter-backing but your saga was so long and drawn out that you have to wonder if regular follow up, starting with good post-op care, would have either nipped it in the bud or at least gotten you to resolution much sooner. He believed that Dr. Rowley brought you in, did the procedure then basically let you go. To him, that was very irresponsible."

"What they did to you was wrong, Kellee," she said, "and I believed right from the beginning that there was no way the experts could not find negligence. I have to say that it really made me angry that these doctors treated you with such callous indifference."

I could tell Ms. Marks was passionate about my case. I could hear the determination in her voice as she talked about what the expert had said. There was no doubt that this woman was definitely on my side. Her voice was the equivalent of the sun penetrating my darkened soul through a bright and shining glass.

"You don't know how long I've wanted to hear someone say what you just said to me," I said, with emotion. "I just could not believe that what these three doctors did to me was right. What really caused me the greatest emotional pain is the thought that they would get away with it."

"Well," Ms. Marks said, "you must always be prepared to expect some hurdles in all medical malpractice litigation. There are very few slam-dunk cases. However, I feel we are at least off to a good start. Are you ready to move on to the Ob/Gyn expert who reviewed Dr. Snyder's aspect of the case?"

"Yes, I am," I replied, trembling with emotion.

"Dr. George Wiest was the Ob/Gyn that reviewed your case," she said. "He said right off the bat that he did not think you were the appropriate candidate for UFE if you were interested in preserving your fertility. He would not have recommended it for you. In fact, if you had brought it up, he would have discouraged you from having it performed. He did not think Dr. Snyder had a lot of knowledge about UFE but he also thought that he has minimal fault in this. He didn't think it would be appropriate for Dr. Snyder to discuss the risks since he really didn't know too much about it. Those risks should have been discussed by Dr. Rowley. He believes the risks that should have been discussed with you were loss of uterus, decrease of ovarian function, and possible infertility as a result of either one of them. He said whomever is performing the procedure is responsible for informing the patient of the risks. Dr. Langford should have informed you of the risks but Dr. Rowley should have gone into more detail.

"Dr. Wiest did not think that the Depo Lupron has an effect on the success or complication rate of UFEs," she continued. "The shot you received prior to the procedure had no effect because it takes up to seven to fourteen days for the Lupron to get in your system. So he didn't think it was involved with the procedure.

"He felt the standard of care for the follow up care after UFE was a difficult question to answer. The reason being is that interventional radiologists do not typically have hospital privileges. His feeling, though, was that they were responsible. He said Dr. Snyder referred you to Dr. Langford and if there is a problem the referring physician is responsible. But he thought Dr. Snyder did the best he could. Dr. Rowley didn't respond to his calls and he believed this was inappropriate."

"Well, Ms. Marks," I interjected, heatedly, "I sure don't agree with him on that point. Dr. Snyder did not do the best he could. I never saw him after he readmitted me to the hospital on May 25th. He turned me over to one of his partners that I had never met with. That was the doctor that discharged me from the hospital, not Dr. Snyder. And he didn't even call me over the six-month period to see how I was doing. He did not answer the nurse's calls while I lay on the gurney in the hallway of Butler Hospital on October 31st. And last but not least, I'll never forget that he 'declined' to come to the hospital on November 1st when I was on my deathbed."

"Kellee, I agree with you," she said. "And please call me Phyllis. Of course this is something that will certainly be brought out before the jury and, believe me, Dr. Snyder's conduct will not look good. But let me finish with Dr. Wiest's opinions.

"He didn't think antibiotics needed to be given," she went on. "He didn't think they are typically given but even if they had been given, the outcome would have been the same because this was necrosis of the uterus, in other words, death of the uterus. He said necrosis of your uterus appeared over a period of several months before it caused complete ischemic infection. Ischemia occurs when the blood supply is cut off to an organ, and in your case, the uterus.

"The bottom line for Dr. Wiest was that you were a patient with a huge uterus and you wanted to preserve your fertility. He thought Dr. Snyder should have considered a myomectomy as an option in your case, although you still could have ended up with a hysterectomy. He believed Dr. Snyder should have laid out all the options to you and clearly explained the risks of each one.

"Dr. Wiest said he thought the interventional radiologists probably wanted experience in doing UFEs," Phyllis said. "It is fairly new in the medical community and they wanted to be able to market UFEs by being the first people to do it, and have the most cases under their belts. Unfortunately, some physicians take inappropriate cases to get that expertise and build up those numbers. That would be his guess as to what occurred in this case.

"It seemed to him that Dr. Snyder was almost roped into this situation by his discussion with Dr. Langford. He may have been looking for an alternative which he felt was in your best interest and, unfortunately, it did not work out that way."

"Well, I sure agree with him on that," I said.

"I'm sure you do," Phyllis responded. "With these opinions from these experts, we feel we are in a position to prepare the affidavit that is required by Georgia law before we can file your medical malpractice case in court," she said. "The affidavit is a sworn statement where the doctor would state what he or she believed to be the acts of negligence engaged in by the doctors. What we want to do before we prepare the affidavits is to wait until we hear from the other two experts. We're very interested in seeing if they will agree with what Dr. Kirby and Dr. Wiest have said."

"When will you hear from them?" I asked.

"I don't think it should be more than a week because it is our practice to set a specific time limit on our experts' review. You know I'll call you as soon as I hear from them but you know you can always call me anytime you have any questions about your case. Joseph is also available if you want to talk to him. One of the things we strongly believe in at this firm is that this is your case and you have a right to know about everything that happens. We work hard to keep out clients informed about their cases. So don't ever hesitate to call us."

"I won't," I said. "You have made my day, Phyllis, and I look forward to hearing from you when you have the information on the other experts."

We said our goodbyes and I hung up the phone.

I didn't know how to feel. There were a myriad of emotions racing through my body. One thing I was sure of was that Phyllis Marks was on fire about my case and that gave me relief beyond belief. I hurried to go tell my mother the good news. Lord knows, she had suffered every painful step of the way with me and I knew this would make her day, too.

When I woke up the next day, my constant companion, Mr. Depression, was back in full force. Yesterday, I was riding on the tide of a mixture of happiness and pleasant disbelief that the experts had reported favorably in my case. Today, I was so angry I could spit nails. I stayed in my bedroom because I did not trust being around anyone in my present state of mind. I was so frantic that I could not stop myself from pacing back and forth across the room.

To find out that I was not the prime candidate for a UFE was a major upset to me. An even bigger shock was finding out that it was *not* common to have six months of pain after the procedure. To think I walked around with my organs necrosing inside me for six months. When I thought back on how hard I had struggled through those six months of pain, trying to save my uterus, I felt like screaming. It was all so unnecessary, because I should never have had the UFE in the first place! I was not even having symptoms from my fibroids! I was beside myself with anger and frustration.

I could not shut Dr. Snyder's and Dr. Langford's voices out of my mind, and their words swirled through my head in a never-ending tormenting cycle: "You're the prime candidate. It's a simple 24-hour outpatient procedure. If you have it done on Friday, you'll be back to work on Monday. It's the miracle cure for fibroids. What's happening to your body is normal post-UFE. You can expect these symptoms to last for up to six months."

I rammed the palms of my hands tightly over my ears in an effort to silence their torturing voices. I had so much rage in my body that I was trembling. I struggled to calm myself down because I knew I was not completely healed from my last hospitalization and this was not good for me. As I felt the pain of my surgical incision, I became so enraged I thought I would explode in a thousand pieces. I had a vision of just punching all three doctors full in the face for all the slick lies they had told me to get me to agree to the procedure. Especially Dr. Snyder because he sealed the deal with Dr. Langford and Dr. Rowley because of the blind trust I placed in him. And to find out he knew diddly-squat about UFEs was too much to bear. Oh! How could he have referred me for a procedure he knew nothing about? Were his patients not important enough for him to at least do some preliminary research about a procedure he was considering referring them for? Or was he just too lazy to bother?

I struggled again to calm myself. I could feel the pain from my recent surgery increasing and I needed to sit down. As I carefully sat down on the bed, I tried to control my breathing. I realized I was so upset I was in danger of hyperventilating. I was crying in deep wracking sobs that hurt my incision and I was holding on to my stomach in an effort to minimize my pain. Huge tears were rolling down my cheeks and my hair was wet from the heat of a hot flash that had hit me in the midst of my distress.

I slowly crawled back into bed and then rolled over on my side. I brought my knees up to my chest so I could relieve the pressure that was causing pain in my abdomen. I was so miserable that I could not stand the daylight and I covered my head with my blankets. I needed complete darkness to confront the blackness I felt in my soul.

True to her word, Phyllis called me about a week later. It had been a rough week for me and although I wanted to hear what the other experts had to say, I knew it would open up the anger wounds again.

"Well, Kellee," she said, "we have the information from the other two experts."

"I hope it's good news," I said. "I had a really rough week. I was glad to hear what the other experts said, but it stirred up my anger issues, big time."

"I knew it would," she said, "but I was hoping the favorable opinions would kind of balance the scales for you in the long run."

"It did, but it just hurts so much to think my life had such little meaning to these doctors," I said, sadly. "I mean, Dr. Snyder didn't even think enough of me to educate himself about a procedure he was referring me for as an alternative treatment for my fibroids. He's the expert and he's supposed to know about everything that has to do with gynecology. At least that's what I thought. I trusted him. I feel so stupid that I did not look into UFEs for myself. You don't know how many times I've beat myself up for not doing this. They have no idea how their cavalier treatment of me as a patient has ruined my life." I was close to tears.

"Kellee," Phyllis said, gently, "you should not blame yourself about this. Most people trust their doctors and most doctors are worthy of their trust. But it's never a bad idea to do your own homework. It's something I encourage people to do whenever I get the chance. That way, when your doctor recommends something for you, you're more prepared to intelligently participate in the decision making process which you should be a part of. I cannot over-stress the importance of taking a proactive stance in your medical care."

"I know that now," I said, wiping the tears from my eyes, "I don't think I'll ever be able to trust doctors again and that makes me feel bad."

"It'll get better as time goes by," she said. "I know it's hard for you to believe that right now, but the process of this case will help to provide some emotional healing for you. How about I tell you what the experts had to say?"

"Okay," I said.

"I'll start again with the interventional radiologist," she said. "This expert's name is Dr. Martin Gunn. He's one of the interventional radiologists that got involved with UFEs early on. In fact, he told me he had done some training seminars for Drs. Langford and Rowley's radiology group. I was somewhat taken aback by that but that really made me interested to know what he had to say or how he trained them."

"Wow! That's quite a coincidence, isn't it?" I asked.

"It is, but not really," she said. "We always try to get the top experts to evaluate our cases so they are usually doctors who have written medical articles on the medical topic we're researching. Oftentimes, we get their names from the articles they've written."

"What did he say?" I could hardly contain my excitement.

"I expected him to be somewhat milder in his criticism of Dr. Langford and Dr. Rowley, since he had something to do with their training, and he was," she said. "His opinion was that it was a matter of judgment as to who is or who is not an appropriate candidate for UFE. Overall, he felt you were probably a proper candidate. Even in the year 2000 he would have still considered a patient interested in preserving her fertility an appropriate candidate. He said that in day-to-day practice it is difficult to weed these people out. Dr. Gunn's response to this question surprised me because all the other experts were not in favor of performing a UFE on women interested in preserving their fertility. When I challenged him on what the medical articles said in reference to not performing UFEs on women interested in fertility, his response was that the authors themselves do not believe that. He said the reason it was stated that way in the article, was because when you write things in articles you don't want people going too far in treating people. So the bottom line was, no, he did not agree with the article the way it was written.

"He really comes across pro-UFE and that's not surprising since he's on the pioneering edge of promoting UFEs. He was quick to point out that the overall chance of hysterectomy after myomectomy is higher than it is after UFE. He says he quotes to his patients that 1 in 200 has a chance of hysterectomy after UFE.

"Dr. Gunn felt that Dr. Snyder had no responsibility in this case and even went so far as to say he should not be named in the suit."

"I'm not liking this doctor's opinions already," I said, cynically.

"I know, but his opinion is not all bad," she said. "Besides, we like to get a good balance from our experts because we really are in search of the true picture. It makes us better prepared for the defendants' experts. To continue, he did not think Dr. Snyder was in a position to discuss UFE in any great detail…"

"Then why did he?" I cried.

"Exactly," she agreed. "We'll be able to address that point at the appropriate time. Dr. Gunn felt it was the responsibility of the interventional radiologist to explain the procedure to the patient. He said Dr. Rowley needed to be sure at the time he performed the UFE that you understood everything. It was his responsibility to explain all the risks and the benefits of UFE."

"Well, he didn't," I said, petulantly.

"I know, and it's our responsibility to prove that, so don't worry about it," she said. "Like the other doctors, he did not feel that your Depo Lupron shot was a contraindication to UFE. He said there was no evidence to show that people on hormone therapy should not be treated. However, he said that interventional radiologists today would not perform a UFE if you had just received a Lupron shot. It is now known that it can restrict the blood vessels to the uterus and fibroids making it difficult to complete this procedure. In 2000, some doctors were just beginning to question whether it should be done."

"I'm beginning to feel more and more like my body was used like a cadaver," I said with amazement.

"I understand your feeling that way," Phyllis said. "I would too if I were in your shoes. On the issue of follow up care, he didn't want to come right out and say that Dr. Rowley was wrong. What he said was that we needed to find out if Dr. Rowley was in town and maybe that's why he wasn't available to answer Dr. Snyder's pages. He did say that if Dr. Rowley was working and he got a couple of phone calls from Dr. Snyder and he did not respond to them, that is not good and in our favor. In general, he said they tell patients how to get in touch with them directly.

"As for the coils, Dr. Gunn said that the coils insure that the uterine arteries are completely blocked. It was felt at that time that it was necessary in order to adequately treat the fibroids and make sure they died or you would have a failed procedure. He said that doctors know now that it is really not necessary but at that time it was the standard of care. It is known now that complete occlusion could have contributed to an injury to the lining of the uterus. This is probably less likely to happen when you do not use coils."

"They used my body as a guinea pig," I said, flatly.

"As I said, I can understand you feeling that way," she said. "His opinion about the antibiotics was the same as the other doctors. He didn't believe it was malpractice not to use them. As to the six month issue, he said flat out he would not agree with such a statement. He said most people would be feeling better sooner. It is rare that patients would have problems beyond one month. In fairness to Dr. Gunn, he did say that if everything is exactly as you said, he thought we have some cause to say you did not get proper informed consent, and you have this sleight of hand switching of doctors which would not look good in front of a jury. He further said, if you never had a follow up conversation with Dr. Rowley that does not meet the standard of care.

"His bottom line was he saw no malpractice as to the technical performance of the UFE. Surprisingly, he thought the follow up care of Dr. Snyder was appropriate," Phyllis said. "He thought the main point of discussion is whether you had a proper informed consent and whether you received adequate care by the interventional radiologists involved in your case.

"Dr. Gunn said you had a terrible complication from the procedure. One of the worse he has heard of. Of course death is worse. But having bowel adhesions is bad. However, Dr. Gunn did not believe that it meant that the doctor who is involved did anything wrong. That is the trouble. Bad things happen when things are done correctly."

"I'll never believe anything was done correctly in my case!" I said, hotly.

"And, obviously, we agree," Phyllis said, as she shuffled some papers. "Let's move on to the Ob/Gyn's opinion, Dr. Alfred Molando. He said right off the bat that most doctors would not offer UFE for a woman who is interested in fertility. So he did not feel you were the best candidate for this procedure. He did not feel there was enough experience with UFE for this question to be answered definitively. He perceived UFE to still be an investigational tool. If a woman says she wants to become pregnant, she should not have this procedure."

My emotions started raging again when I heard this but I said nothing for fear I would lose control and just start bawling. I could feel prickly sensations all over my body.

"Dr. Molando felt that Dr. Rowley should have counseled you about the risks more than Dr. Snyder," she continued. "He said nobody really knows the role of the gynecologist or the role of the interventional radiologist in terms of counseling. It was his opinion though that both should counsel the patient thoroughly. The gynecologist is not the radiologist, and the radiologist is not the gynecologist. From some aspect they must work together in order to deliver the best care. He thought there was a problem in that regard. He felt that Dr. Snyder should definitely have explained the side effects of UFE to you. Especially for someone wanting to preserve her fertility, which of course you did. He did not believe UFE should be offered to this patient. He commented that interventional radiologists send patients to him for consultation before performing a UFE.

"Dr. Molando agreed with Dr. Kirby in that he did not believe the Lupron shot had a chance to do anything in the very short course that it was there," Phyllis went on. "For it to have had an effect in two to three days was very unlikely. He said he did not think there is a consensus among doctors about how to handle Lupron.

"As to the follow up care, Dr. Molando said if you do a procedure, you should be responsible and be around for complications," she said. "The interventional radiologist wants the Gyn to be available because you can have necrosis and have to do an emergency hysterectomy. The interventional radiologist cannot do this and that is why they have to work together to do the best they can for their patients. He said the physicians should have communicated better and someone should have been available at all times. When you perform the procedure you must be available for the patient.

"He felt that most doctors do not use coils but that it is not a mistake," she stated. "He did not believe the coils were a strong point for us even though most doctors will not use them. He also said that doctors in his hospital use antibiotics but you don't have to. The death of the uterus is not from infection but rather the result of the decrease in blood supply of the uterine wall that results in necrosis and death of the wall of the uterus.

"As to switching physicians, he does not believe it is right for one physician to speak to the patient and then another physician performs the procedure," she said. "He felt this was unacceptable. He believed it was important for the patient to know her physician and he is the one who should take the consent. And the patient should accept this physician to perform the surgery. He felt this was a breach of trust between the physician and the patient. He believed you should have met Dr. Langford face-to-face because it is inappropriate to do a consultation over the phone. Certainly when it involves an investigational tool, a modality that has not been totally explored. Complications are involved. And certainly not to someone who wants to become pregnant.

"Dr. Molando felt Dr. Rowley's unavailability is another strong point. He believed that if this could be documented based on your medical records, it could not be defended in court. If you do a procedure you have to be available for complications. He definitely thought there was room for improvement here. He felt that when you take care of a patient and certainly when you perform a procedure, you must be around for the patient. There is no other way around it.

"In a nutshell, Dr. Molando felt that Ob/Gyns have to be very careful when they offer this investigational treatment. He believes the gynecologist must be involved in the care of these patients even though he is not the one performing the UFE. Before he sends his patients to an expert, he has to be involved in her care. He tells her everything that he knows about it and even gives her his article to read. He has a session in the office with his patient where she can ask him questions. He tells her if he thinks the procedure is right for her. Only then, would he send her to an interventional radiologist.

"That about wraps it up, Kellee. Now we'll have the experts sign the affidavits I told you about and we'll file your case in court. As I said, this is not a slam-dunk case but we do believe we have some issues to fight with. We'll keep you posted as we move along. I'm going to have to go now but if you find you have any questions, feel free to call me back. Okay?"

"Sure, Phyllis," I said. "I really appreciate everything you've done and even though this is painful for me, I do feel much better knowing the truth. I know it will take time for me to get through this."

"I agree," she said. "Call me anytime you need to." She said goodbye and hung up.

Well, I thought at least we're off to the races. I could finally relax now that I knew a lawsuit was going to be filed in my behalf. I was glad I did not give up when Mr. Matheson told me I didn't have a case. I felt somewhat vindicated.

If I thought the worst was behind me in terms of dirty little secrets, the worst was yet to come.

Chapter Eight

And the Plot Thickens

Used as a guinea pig. Used like a cadaver! These thoughts reverberated in my mind over the next few months after talking to Phyllis. From what I had heard, it was obvious that none of the three doctors was well-versed in UFEs, period. Dr. Langford had been so glib during the phone conversation he had with me when he helped to convince me I was the prime candidate. He had obviously learned the proper buzz words in order to get Dr. Snyder to donate my so trusting body to his radiology group for experimentation. It was not necessary for us to talk for that long because Dr. Snyder had already sealed the deal for him.

During this conversation he neglected to tell me that UFE was a so-called investigational tool. They can call it "investigational" all they want but the bottom line is they experimented on me. They neglected to tell me all of the risks associated with UFE. No one never ever discussed any alternative treatments. No doubt about it, Dr. Langford's radiology group wanted a warm body to experiment on so they could get some notches on their belts so it would make it easier for them to go after more unsuspecting victims. And then Dr. Langford had the nerve to shift me over to one of his partners without my authorization or consent. I still could not get over that. No doubt about it, these guys were practicing bootleg medicine.

All three doctors were poor representations for the medical profession. In my opinion, it is these kind of doctors that give good doctors a bad name. Even though I had been fortunate to have excellent doctors for my heart surgery, the treatment of Drs. Snyder, Langford, and Rowley was so heartless that it had seriously damaged my ability to trust doctors like I did before. I had certainly been taken in by Dr. Snyder. How do you weed out the good doctors from the bad ones? I would never have dreamed Dr. Snyder would treat a patient so abominably. So how would I ever know who was real from who was Memorex?

Unquestionably, I was grateful for the doctors that saved my life after the UFE. Yet I could not help but feel resentment toward them for not being truthful with me. How could it be possible for Dr. Thomas to not have known what happened to me, if he was the gynecologist that operated on me and saw the mess that was created from my UFE? It was clear that he was in no way going to criticize Dr. Snyder. And to think he suggested that I go back to Dr. Snyder for a follow up visit after witnessing the mutilation inside my body. I adored Dr. Olson, yet he would not tell me what really happened to me, either. It was as though they were all covering up for the doctors that nearly killed me, with their indifference and negligence. It was a hard pill to swallow.

Phyllis had put it bluntly. "Kellee," she had said, "what you have to understand is that it is rare for a doctor to say anything critical about another doctor's treatment, no matter how bad it is. In fairness to them, if they do make statements, they could find themselves in the center of a lawsuit and they certainly don't want that. There is definitely a conspiracy of silence among doctors and, as a group they are very good at watching each others' back. They'll close ranks on you in a heartbeat. That's just the way it is. But then again, that's one of the reasons medical malpractice has evolved to such increased proportions over the last twenty years. Patients who have been injured resent this."

I smiled when I thought of Phyllis. She was definitely my hero. She was so passionate about my case that now I knew she had been given the fire I lost. I spoke with her on several occasions and she somehow knew exactly what to say to fix whatever it was that was bothering me. She really listened to me. Numerous times I found myself holding the receiver, speechless. What was she? A psychic with a law degree? Every time I spoke with her I knew she truly understood my emotional pain.

I finally met Phyllis, in person, one day in late May 2002. I had to come to the office to sign some papers and we finally saw each other face-to-face. I was not surprised by how she looked. Her physical appearance was a perfect match with the personality that came across so strongly over the phone. She had a presence about her that was quite striking and she would always stand out in a crowd. Phyllis was a little powerhouse of a woman, beautiful and strong. She had an air of fearless determination about her. She may have been small in stature but she was tall in character and grace. She embraced me as though she had known me all of her life. Her smile was beautiful and I was instantly comfortable with her. She had just come back from New York.

"It's so good to finally meet you in person, Kellee," she said, beaming at me. She had large sensitive brown eyes that were intelligent and intense. Her short-cropped hair was very becoming to her total look that reeked of class and style.

"It's good to finally see you to!" I said, as I sat down in the chair in front of her desk.

For the next thirty minutes we chatted like we were old friends who had not seen each other in ages. She was genuinely interested in how I had been doing since my last surgery. I did not want to talk about that too long because it stirred up too many emotions. I wanted this to be a pleasant visit without me becoming emotional and spoiling my good mood.

"So we have my case all filed now?" I asked.

"Yes," she said, dramatically rolling her eyes toward the ceiling. "I had to go to New York to get Dr. Molando's affidavit signed. We couldn't file your lawsuit without it. We needed his, along with Dr. Kirby's affidavit. He's extremely busy and we got so close to your filing deadline that Joseph and I didn't want to risk it coming through the mail and maybe getting lost. So I hopped a plane and went and got it. It was a one-day trip and I was pooped by the time I got back."

"Wow," I said. "That's real dedication to do something like that."

"Well, we couldn't allow anything bad to happen to your case," she said, "so I did what I had to do."

"What happens next?" I asked.

Phyllis leaned back in her chair, and assumed a relaxed and comfortable position. "All three doctors will have thirty days to answer the complaint and then the discovery period begins. Discovery is where we get to investigate all aspects of the case. During this period we send out interrogatories to gather more information about the doctors. Interrogatories are questions we ask that will help us to prepare for the doctors' depositions when we're ready to take them. Discovery is also the period where the doctors get to investigate our side too. Which means they will get to send questions to you too so they can prepare for when they take your deposition."

"I'm not looking forward to that," I said. "What can I expect?"

"They can ask you questions about yourself," she answered. "They'll want to know your background and will be assessing how you would appear before a jury if the case should go all the way to trial. They'll surely ask you very detailed questions about what you remember happening with the doctors. Sometimes, after taking the deposition of the plaintiff, defense attorneys might decide to settle the case and then it doesn't go to trial."

"Do you think my case will settle before going to trial?" I asked. "I sure hope so."

"It's hard to make that call right now," she replied. "There are too many things that are unknown. We'll know more when we get the answers to the complaint and especially when we get answers to our interrogatories. The interrogatory answers will tell us a lot because we draft them to get specific information."

"Like what do you think would be important?" I asked.

"For one thing," she said, "we'll be very interested to know how many UFEs Dr. Langford and Dr. Rowley have performed prior to your procedure in May 2000. My guess is that they have not performed very many. We're really looking forward to finding out that information. We'll also want to know about any conversations they recall having with you and what the details of those conversations were. That kind of information."

"Well, I sure will be interested to know the answers to all those questions," I sighed. "I can't get the thought out of my mind that they callously used my body like a cadaver."

"We'll certainly find out if they did," she said. "The whole point of interrogatories is to ferret out the answers that will help to strengthen our case."

We sat and talked for a little longer and then Phyllis stood up to walk me to the elevator. As we walked out of her office, she said she wanted me to meet the other people in the law firm so I would be familiar with everybody. They were a small firm so everyone knew about my case and were in some way involved in it. We passed by Joseph's office so I stuck my head in and waved and said, "Hi."

Further along the way, she introduced me to the other members of the law firm.

"This is Alice Stevens, the business manager for the firm," she said, as we stood in the doorway of Alice's office. "Alice this is Kellee Kendell. Alice is the one who keeps up with all the expenses for your case so you'll want to know her," Phyllis said jokingly. Alice stood up and came around her desk to shake my hand. She was a sweet and motherly looking woman. "Hi Kellee," she said with a warm smile, "it's nice to finally meet you." Her eyes were a penetrating blue and they sparkled with intelligence.

Walking out of Alice's office, we walked a few steps to Sandra Thorpe's work area. She was the paralegal. She pulled the Dictaphone plugs out of her ears as we were introduced. "Hi Kellee," she said and shook my hand. "I've typed up a lot of letters dictated for you," she laughed. I laughed too.

I had such a warm feeling about this law firm. Everyone was so genuine and down to earth, including Joseph. They were definitely the essence of a close-knit family. The receptionist had gone to lunch.

Standing in front of the elevators, Phyllis said, "You take care of yourself, Kellee," as she gave me a warm hug. "We'll keep you posted on how your case is going. Of course if you have any questions, you know you can call us anytime."

I stepped into the elevator and said goodbye.

The next several months were hard on me. My emotions were like a roller-coaster, up and down, up and down. I could not seem to pull myself out of my depression. The Paxil was starting to help, but I still lived in constant fear of another bowel obstruction that might land me back in the hospital. I still felt pains in my stomach and this made me think the adhesions were growing again in my abdomen. I had not been able to get off my diet of daily pain pills. I'd never gotten my energy back from my emergency surgeries, and I began to be afraid that I would never get my real estate career up and running again.

I felt so guilty that my mother had to help me out financially now. I know my circumstances were a financial drain on her and it made me feel really bad. Still, I was too afraid to leave Ohio and go back home to Atlanta. What if something happened to me and I got sick again? Would I get to the hospital in time? And I cringed when I thought of Kendell ever again having to go through watching paramedics put me into an ambulance, and then being left alone. Although he was a mature teenager for fourteen, he had been traumatized by that experience. I'll never forget the fear I saw in my son's eyes.

I struggled daily with anger issues. No matter how hard I tried to put it all behind me, I just could not get over the senselessness of it all. To have gone through all I went through and I was never sick in the first place, was just too much for me to deal with. I tormented myself by asking over and over, "Why didn't I listen to my mother?"

My mother had suffered through this every step of the way and it had taken its toll on her. I could see new fine lines in her face from all the worry she had endured at my expense. She seemed to be more tired these days and I knew her constant anxiety about me having another attack drained her of her usually vibrant energy. When I saw the tremendous impact my illness had on my mother, it made me loathe the doctors who did this to me. I was sure that they had gone on with their lives as though I never even existed. I'll bet they did not miss a step and that I was some vague memory in the far recesses of their minds as they went about enjoying life in a way I could not. It seemed so unfair. For the first time I had some insight into why people could go postal.

I had heard many times that life was not fair but I never thought it would get this bad. I was not naive enough to think that hard times would not come my way and I knew that I was not exempt from challenges in my life. However, this took the cake. And all over fibroids that were not even giving me any trouble. It all seemed too cruel.

The thought that these doctors would get away with their negligent treatment of me was a thought I absolutely could not tolerate. To think that they would not in some way be held accountable for what they did to me was enough to send me into a blue funk for hours. It was just not right. Besides, what if they did this to some other woman? Had they done this to other women? Were there other women out there who had gone through the same hellish experience as I did from a UFE? I wondered.

When the summer rolled into late August, I got a call from Phyllis.

I answered the phone and she said, "Kellee, this is Phyllis Marks. Is this a good time to talk to you?"

"Oh yes," I said.

"Well," she said, "we've received some answers to our interrogatories. Are you sitting down? If you're not, I want you to sit down."

I could hear some tension in Phyllis's voice. I could hear her breathing over the phone. I felt the pressure of fear grip my entire chest area as I sat down. "I'm sitting down," I said weakly.

She hurried and said, "We asked Drs. Langford and Rowley how many UFEs they had performed before your procedure in May 2000. Dr. Langford had performed none and Dr. Rowley had performed one." Phyllis stopped talking. There was complete silence on the phone as I absorbed this shock.

Finally, she said, "Kellee, I'm so angry I don't know what to do. I never in my wildest imagination thought that Dr. Langford had not performed *any* UFEs at the time he talked you into getting one. I'm angry that he didn't tell you he had never performed the procedure before. You deserved to know that and also that the procedure was investigational and something new for the treatment of fibroids. I consider it an experimental procedure no matter what they choose to call it. I'm incensed. I resent the use of the word 'investigational' when in fact it's clearly experimental. Doctors use this play on words because if they say the procedure is experimental that would scare a lot of women away from them making a $7,500 fee for a forty-five minute procedure. Some doctors probably charge even more."

I could hear the outrage in her voice. "And to think that Dr. Rowley had only performed one UFE before performing yours," she said disbelievingly. "You were right all along—they did use you as a guinea pig. Actually, cadaver is more appropriate because you're a human being, not an animal. Only you were alive at the time. I'm really quite shocked and I have to tell you, I didn't think it would be this bad. You're lucky to have escaped with your life."

I was still speechless on the other end of the line. I could feel tears starting to form in my eyes but I was determined not to cry. Oddly, I became concerned about Phyllis being so upset.

"I knew all along they were incompetent," I said, struggling to keep my composure. "I at least had the right to know the extent of their experience. It hurts so bad that I trusted Dr. Snyder and he turned me over to, not one, but two inexperienced doctors. I just can't get over the fact that he would be so careless in his referrals."

"There's more, Kellee," she said. "Dr. Langford claims that he discussed the procedure with you in detail and answered your questions. He said he discussed your symptoms, how the procedure was performed, and alternative treatments such as medical and surgical therapy, the potential complications and risks of the procedure, its effect on fertility and the advantages and disadvantages of the UFE procedure, among other things."

"That's a flat out lie!" I cried. "The only thing Dr. Langford said was that it was a simple 24-hour outpatient procedure! He said exactly what Dr. Snyder said to me. We never talked about any symptoms because I didn't have any. He never said there would be *any* complications or risks. I will never forget what he said because it almost cost me my life. If he had told me anything at all about risks, I never would have had it done. I'm a previous open heart surgery patient. Would it make sense for me to take any risks with my body? The way he described it was like something no more complicated than getting a tooth pulled. Maybe two days of discomfort and then everything would be fine. He never ever said anything about fertility. Why is he lying like this?"

"Because it's not in his best interest to tell the truth," Phyllis answered. "If he told the truth it would be the equivalent of admitting his negligence. I'm sure he's been advised of this by his lawyers and they know it's our job to prove that he didn't say all those things to you. They know it boils down to a he-said-she-said scenario and they're banking on a jury that would believe doctors are incapable of telling lies."

"Well they are," I said heatedly. I was so angry I was trembling. That sick feeling in the pit of my stomach was back in full force and I was starting to feel queasy. "What did Dr. Rowley say?" I was almost afraid to ask.

"He pretty much said the same thing," she answered. "He said he introduced himself to you as the physician who would be performing the procedure, explained the procedure, apologized for the delay, and asked you if you had any questions about the procedure. He also said he spoke with you the day after and asked you how you were feeling. He said he had a conversation with your mother."

"I don't believe this!" I cried. "I wouldn't know Dr. Rowley from Adam's house-cat! I have no idea what he looks like. For that matter, I have no idea what either one of them looks like. If I saw them on the street I wouldn't know who they were!"

"I know this is upsetting to you, Kellee," Phyllis said. "I have to admit I'm somewhat taken aback by all this myself. But remember that it's our job to bring out the true facts. I'm not surprised that they would lie about what they told you. What I am surprised about is that they had no experience. I'm, quite frankly, flabbergasted."

"What will you do now?" I asked.

"We'll go forward with setting up a time to get all the doctors' depositions now that we have the answers to their interrogatories," she answered. "Don't you worry about it Kellee because you know we'll be doing everything in our power at this law firm to bring out the truth. I hated to call you and tell you this but as I've said from the beginning, this is your case and you have the right to know everything that's going on in it. Besides, I knew you'd want to know."

"I would want to know, but I still can't believe that they would lie like this," I said, feeling like all the wind had been knocked out of me. "I guess I've lived in a world of Peter Pan and the Easter Bunny because I never thought the lies would be this extreme. They know they're lying."

"I believe they are lying," she agreed, "but we've got to be able to prove it. Unfortunately, that's the name of the game. I don't want you to make yourself sick worrying about this. This is how cases go and we have to position ourselves on how we can best respond to what they've said. You know you're telling the truth and I really believe a jury will know that too if we have to go to trial."

"How will we ever be able to prove they're lying?" I asked, the fear evident in my voice.

"I haven't figured it out yet, but I want you to know I won't give up trying," she said with fierce determination. "I'm really doing in-depth research into this whole area surrounding uterine fibroids and UFE. I'm finding some very intriguing information. When I've completed more of this process, I'll share my findings with you. Right now I've got to go but I wanted to call you and tell you about this as soon as I knew."

We said a few more words and then I hung up the phone.

I sat there, frozen in shock over what I'd just heard. As awareness continued to overtake me, I felt my body begin to percolate with a dangerous rage. However, it was an impotent rage and I was in a frenzy trying to find an outlet for it. I wanted more than anything in the world to see these doctors brought to justice but now I saw that it was going to be a long and tortuous road. There would be no comfort for me until my mission was accomplished, to this end. The thought that I could be so callously experimented on stuck in my craw and I knew I would never be able to let this go. No matter what the outcome of my case, I would find a way to expose this kind of medical treachery.

Propelled by my anger, I reached down into the depths of my soul and ripped out the strength I needed to take me through what I knew would be the most difficult journey of my life. I pushed aside the sickness and pain that had dogged my footsteps and stolen the spirit of determination, resolve, and fearlessness I once possessed. I resolutely willed my body to knit itself back together from the mammoth mutilation, destruction, and abuse that was wreaked on it by three avariciously motivated doctors. You can do it! my mind shouted.

With determination, I threw my shoulders back and sat up straight. I felt the fight coming back into my body. What could I do to let the world know what the medical profession's finest was capable of? What could I do to let women know how dangerous it is to trust their doctors, unconditionally? Oprah needs to know about this! I raged. She would surely want to have this travesty of medical injustice aired on her show. If I had to, I would go on every talk show I could to let the truth of my story be known. Somehow I believed I would be embraced by ABC, CBS, and NBC. I had no idea how I was going to do this but the warrior blood was beginning to pump strongly through my veins.

Impelled by a flash of insight born of desperation, I bolted out of the chair and ran upstairs to my bedroom. I shot through the door like one possessed and retrieved the pain medication and Paxil from my bedside stand. In a rush, I popped the child-proof caps off the bottles and dashed toward the bathroom before I could even think about changing my mind. Gripping a medication bottle in each hand, I bent over and frantically shook the pills into the toilet, delighting in the plopping sounds they made as they hit the water. I stood up straight. I turned and flung the empty bottles into the trash can, then whipped around and pushed down, hard, on the handle, and flushed the toilet. I stood watching as the pills swirled in a fast-flowing circle and then disappeared under the pressure of the water. Now, I thought, my mind will be clear and sharp, unhampered by the dullness that overcame me as a result of taking these pills.

I stood even taller. I had been beaten down, but like the phoenix, I had risen from the burning ashes of my ruin, renewed. I had become a powerful foe to be reckoned with. Gone was the weak and frightened wraith of a person I had been reduced to by the negligent treatment of three doctors. In the weaklings place, stood an eight-foot sword-wielding Amazon, fearless, strong, and ready to kick ass.

I resolved that Phyllis would not go into battle alone. I would not let these doctors defeat me no matter what. They had lied but I was determined they would not get away with it. They had back-pedaled like two mad dogs trying to avoid stepping in their own vomit. Now, that was an interesting play on words considering how much vomit *I'd* had to tolerate over the last fifteen months. No sir, their conduct would not go unanswered by me.

I was still riding this tide of heightened furor when Phyllis called me back a few days later. Even before I answered the phone, I somehow knew it was her. I snatched the receiver and said, "Hello?"

"Hey, Kellee," she said, "this is Phyllis. How are you today?"

"Oh, I'm much better, thanks," I said. "I was knocked for a loop after our last phone conversation but I'm back. What's going on?" I asked.

"You know I told you I was doing some in-depth research over the Internet in the area of fibroids and UFEs. Well, I've found some interesting things, I must say," she said, sounding pleased with herself.

"Really?" I said. "I'm all ears."

She continued. "It's amazing how much information there is on the Internet about this subject. It's also amazing how conflicting the information is. I came across a web-site that was set up by the HERS foundation which is an independent non-profit international women's health organization. They have a link to uterine fibroid embolization. Actually they called it uterine artery embolization on their web-site and I'll explain later what the difference is. I found it interesting that the first thing that was said was, 'With the extremely rapid popularization of Uterine Artery Embolization it is important for the public to have access to the known effects of this new surgery.' From what is said on this site, there is no question that UFE is being rapidly promoted and popularized but I thought it was good that this organization has come right out and put the known adverse effects, right up front."

"That is good," I agreed. "What did the HERS site say about UFE?"

"It said that UFE was experimental, invasive, exposed the ovaries, uterus and vagina to radiation, and that it is unreliable," she answered with obvious glee. "It listed the adverse effects that have also been reported in the medical publications. I've run across of lot of them during the course of my research. They listed death, infection, misembolization, ovarian damage, loss of ovarian function, infertility, can you believe that?" she exclaimed.

"That sure isn't what the Three Stooges told me," I said. "Well, actually Dr. Rowley didn't tell me anything."

"They sure didn't tell you any of this," she agreed. "They list even more effects. Loss of orgasm is another effect. I tell you I'd be really be ticked-off about that one!" she laughed. "It's really no joking matter though because these things can really happen from UFEs. There can be failure of the embolization surgery, menopause, Post-Embolization Syndrome (PES), now this sounds like what happened in your case. PES is characterized by acute and/or chronic pain. Remember how you ran those high temperatures?" she asked.

"How could I ever forget," I said derisively.

"I know," she said. "Women with PES can have temperatures up to 102 degrees. And I know this is going to get to you; it is also characterized by depression, nausea, vomiting, and severe night sweats."

"I don't believe any of this!" I exclaimed. "How is it that this is on a web-site that has nothing to do with doctors and they know about PES and the Three Stooges didn't?" I asked. I was beginning to delight in this characterization of the three doctors who had irreparably harmed my body. They deserved no better since they had rendered incompetent and lackadaisical treatment to me. Actually, it was more like mis-treatment and no-treatment.

"Well," she answered," I found this enlightening too. If Dr. Snyder had bothered to do a tiny bit of research he would have discovered this. It sure didn't take me long to find this web site. It just goes to show you how indifferent and lazy Dr. Snyder was. I'll bet he wouldn't want anyone treating his wife in this uncaring manner."

"I know," I said.

"They certainly treated you in an extremely shoddy fashion. I think veterinarians would have more concern and regard for their dogs than these doctors had for you," Phyllis said huffily.

"You're not kidding about that!" I exclaimed.

"There are even more adverse effects listed," she continued. "Hysterectomy…"

"Oh, my God," I could not help but interrupt. "And to think Dr. Snyder had the nerve to tell me UFE was the sure way to *avoid* hysterectomy."

"I know, Kellee," she said sympathetically, "but there are still more adverse side effects listed. Severe persistent pain, hematoma, vaginal discharge containing pus and blood, bleeding from the incision site, fibroid expulsion, which is fibroids pushing out through the vagina…"

"Ugh!" I could not help interrupting again. "That sounds really gross! I'll bet if women knew about that they would really think hard before having a UFE."

"Yes," she agreed, "but even grosser is *unsuccessful* fibroid expulsion where the fibroid becomes trapped in the cervix causing infection and requiring surgical removal. You know that's got to cause a tremendous amount of pain because even when a blood clot gets trapped during a woman's menstrual period that hurts like hell."

"I know," I said, reeling from the shock of it all.

"And still there's more," she continued. "Life threatening allergic reaction to the contrast medium can occur too and, last but not least, uterine adhesions." Phyllis paused and gave me time for this to sink in.

And it did. Incredible. All I had suffered had been known adverse effects all along. It was unconscionable that none of the doctors bothered to mention these things to me. It had to be intentional unless they were so dumb they didn't know about the adverse effects, and I found this hard to believe. They had blatantly lied. There was nothing simple about this procedure.

She continued. "The HERS site further indicates that the long term effects of the polyvinyl alcohol particles that they shoot up into the uterine arteries are not known at this time. There has to be a lot more research and time for that research to take place before many questions can be answered definitively. Ironically, the site pointed out that this "unknown" status was also used to describe the early introduction of a number of women's treatment which later proved to be disastrous. Some examples are diethylstilbestrol (DES) which was given to prevent miscarriage and it was ultimately found not to prevent miscarriage but to lead to breast cancer in many of the women who took it. It also caused vaginal cancers and infertility in the daughters they gave birth to, and testicular cancer and infertility in their sons."

"This is terrible," I said, "how is it that the FDA allows this to happen? I thought it was supposed to prevent these kinds of medical atrocities from happening."

"I know," she said, "but sometimes the medical issues that come before the FDA can be very political and driven by selfish interests of big corporations or as, in this case, doctors. I'll be getting to the FDA in a minute. The other catastrophes that have occurred in women under this "unknown" status are the intrauterine device (IUD) which caused life-threatening pelvic infection, infertility, and hysterectomy in many women. Also, silicone breast implants are a part of this group where it was later found that the silicone implants may lead to autoimmune disease. And really sad is, Thalidomide, which was given to pregnant women and caused the babies to be malformed and born with incomplete or missing limbs. Are you beginning to see how dangerous "unknown" statuses can be? That's exactly what's going on with UFEs because the long-term effects are unknown. And they think that as long as they call it "investigational" that makes everything okay. But even admitting that it's investigational should cast healthy suspicion on UFEs. That shows very clearly why they stay way away from calling it "experimental" and will fight tooth and nail to keep that labeling off of it. The truth is that long term effects can only emerge over time and before doctors go off half-cocked promoting UFEs as the be-all and end-all for uterine fibroids, there's still a lot of independent research that needs to be done."

"I'm just in a state of shock," I managed to say. "It's just too much but I'm really glad I'm hearing this."

"I know I've dropped a lot on you today but I do want to cover one more thing I think would be of interest to you and that is the Fibroid Registry," she continued. "The first thing that I find of interest about the Fibroid Registry is that it is owned and operated by the Cardiovascular and Interventional Radiology Research Foundation. Of course, interventional radiologists are the doctors who would benefit most from this procedure being approved by the FDA. I see this as a serious conflict."

"I do too," I said, "Dr. Langford and Dr. Rowley are interventional radiologists."

"Exactly," she agreed. "The Registry is supposedly set up for the purpose of collecting information that will be helpful to research about UFEs. The doctors who participate in the Registry are supposed to submit all data regarding relevant cases performed under their sponsorship. They have a long list of requirements for doctors to become participants of the Registry, however, it doesn't say anything about doctors not being permitted to perform this procedure if they are not members of the Registry. I, quite frankly, don't see how that makes any sense. Participating doctors are supposed to get an informed patient consent before they can use the patient's information on the Registry site."

"Wait a minute!" I exclaimed, excited. "A nurse called me from Drs. Langford and Rowley's office. At least I think she was a nurse."

"When did that happen?" Phyllis asked.

"I'm not sure exactly when, but I know it was a little over a year after I had my UFE," I answered. "I remember her telling me something about a Fibroid Registry. I do know I told this woman all the negative things that happened to me and she was very surprised. The thing I remember the most is her being surprised that I did not get antibiotics prior to the procedure. I told her I had not had any symptoms prior to the procedure, and I recall specifically telling her I had no pain or heavy bleeding. She told me that she wanted to discuss this with the doctors and get back with me. I never heard from her again."

"Um," Phyllis said, "that's very interesting. Probably, when she told the doctors what you said about all that had gone wrong, I'm sure the last thing they wanted to do was report your case to the Registry. The truth is, your case was never reported to the Registry, which I find reprehensible. I'm sure you would have been more than happy to sign the consent form. How can the Registry gather the accurate data about UFEs if the doctors can pick and choose which cases they want to submit? And there is no mandatory requirement that interventional radiologists have to be a participant of the Registry *before* they can perform UFEs.

"I'm thinking about all this and it's really making me mad," I said angrily. "It just gets worse and worse. And the FDA accepts this?"

"Apparently it does because from what I can see, the FDA is all poised to approve UFE as an alternative treatment for uterine fibroids," she said. "I read the transcript from the FDA UAE (UFE) meeting on May 22, 2001. That's where the doctors submitted the data they had collected, in an effort to persuade the FDA that UFE should be approved as an alternative treatment. As a matter of fact, one of the experts that reviewed your case, Dr. Gunn, was one of the presenters before the FDA. Of course, the negative aspects of UFEs was treated very mildly. As I told you before, Dr. Gunn is really pro-UFE. You have to remember that UFEs can be pretty lucrative at $7,500 or more a procedure. And what doctors charge is at their discretion.

"You don't have to tell me," I said with disgust. "I learned first hand about that."

Phyllis said, "From what I read, I could tell the FDA appeared to be very receptive to what Dr. Gunn was saying. "The reason I say this is because I read an interesting portion in the transcript of the meeting that included the presentation, by phone, of a Dr. Myra Lofton and the panel didn't have one single response or any questions for her. Needless to say, this doctor was against UFE and in favor of more research before approval. The other thing I found interesting is that is was openly stated in the meeting by a Dr. Donald Singleton, who concluded his presentation by saying that the meeting before the FDA had been a large effort from the Society, i.e. interventional radiologists."

"What did Dr. Lofton have to say?" I asked, curious.

"I have to tell you I truly admired her spunk to have come out so strongly against UFEs in a meeting where it was obvious that the deck was clearly stacked against her," Phyllis answered. "Right off the bat she told the panel that she was an extremely biased and extremely opinionated individual when it came to UFE. She said that the general destruction of normal uterine tissue is the result of uterine artery embolization. Imagine that! Of course, the interventional radiologists have changed the name from uterine artery embolization to uterine fibroid embolization because it speaks more to what they're trying to target. But the truth of the matter is that it's the uterine arteries that are being embolized, not the fibroids."

"I can see where UFE would be a much more powerful marketing tool than UAE," I commented.

"Yes," Phyllis agreed. "Dr. Lofton expressed her distress to hear in the meeting that, after the fact, 10,000 UFE cases had already been performed *before* the Fibroid Registry was set up. She told the FDA about 10 patients who all had very bad outcomes with UFE and that these 10 patients were never reported to the FDA, or followed up."

"I knew it! I knew it!" I practically screamed. "I've always believed there were more women out there who had suffered bad results just like me!"

"Well, you're absolutely right, according to Dr. Lofton, " she agreed. "Dr. Lofton gave the FDA a lot of medical data during her presentation. The thing I found to be the most profound, in reference to our case, is her declaration that all the negatives of UFE are *not* being discussed with the patients. She expressed great concerns over the lack of adequate informed consent. She also expressed concern that there was so much silence on this point. She asked the FDA why the case of a Mildred Duncan was never reported to the FDA because this woman apparently had incredibly disastrous results from UFE. She pointed out again that ten women had reported major complications and that these women had never been reported to the FDA."

"Well," I said, "they sure never reported my case to the Fibroid Registry. That nurse never called me back from Dr. Rowley's office. I guess they only wanted good UFE outcomes to report."

"I feel you," she said. "Dr. Lofton also pointed out that the marketing aspect of UFE is enormous and that's true from what I can see. They're pushing UFE, hard, everywhere and depicting it in just way they described it to you. A wonderful alternative for fibroids."

"Not a 'wonderful alternative,'" I pointed out, "they made it sound like a miracle cure for fibroids."

"Well," she said, "they're not going quite that far in their marketing statements."

"The Three Stooges did," I cried.

"Yes, they did," Phyllis said, laughing at my depiction of the three doctors. "Well, Miss Kellee, I think I've given you enough to think about for one session. It was quite a lot, don't you think?

"Yes I do," I answered, "but it has all been quite enlightening to me. The pieces to the puzzle are finally coming together for me. Now when I ask myself the question 'why' I know some of the answers. It's a relief to be coming out of the dark where I didn't know anything and the doctors wouldn't tell me anything either. I was so frustrated. I always knew they did something wrong, though."

"Yes, you've said that all along," she said. "Kellee there's one more thing I wanted to tell you. We need to get some dates from you and your mother. Opposing counsel want to set up your depositions."

"What!" I exclaimed. "Why do they want my mother's deposition? She's already been to hell and back from all this."

"As I told you before, we're in the discovery phase and they have the right to request depositions from all relevant parties," she replied. "Your mother was a witness to a lot of the things you went through so they want to find out what she knows."

"It just never ends," I sighed. "I'll call you back with some dates. My mom has to come all the way from Ohio so I can't expect her to just drop everything and come down to Atlanta. I'll want to talk with you about what to expect from the depositions but I'm just too mentally exhausted right now."

"I understand," she said. "I'll look to hear from you when you can get some dates arranged. As always, call me if you have any questions about anything."

We hung up the phone.

I sat in the same spot for a while just letting everything seep into my brain. I rubbed the sides of my throbbing temples. It had been so much to digest but I was glad to have some light shed on this subject that had been dark for so long. I was grateful to Phyllis for being so thorough in her research.

It occurred to me that shining the light into dark corners can sometimes cause rats to come scurrying out of the woodwork. Considering their incredible lack of foresight, maybe a more appropriate name for the Three Stooges would be the Three Blind Mice.

Chapter Nine

Facing My Demons

I had run to Atlanta in 1989. I had run to Naples in 1999 and then back to Atlanta in 2000. You can run but you sure can't hide. I do not know where this aphorism comes from but it is definitely true. I had heard it all my life but never paid much attention to it. I was too busy running to stop and smell the coffee, flowers, or anything else. During the course of my ten-year sprint, I had pulled myself up by my bootstraps and could stand tall and proud in any crowd. I had set a course for myself that would shrivel the will of the faint at heart, but I was strong and fearless. Failure was not an option.

But, the year 2000 had brought me up short and stopped me dead in my tracks. I was struck like lightening by foes that hit me head-on, lifted my body twenty feet in the air, and then slam-dunked me onto the side of a stubborn unyielding mountain. Looking up from the ground, flat on my back, I at first did not know what had hit me. Then I realized I had been sucker-punched by three doctor-foes who were equipped with a fully supplied army worthy of Attila the Hun. In their arsenal of weapons of body destruction, they carried deception, the appearance of respectability, ignorance, slothfulness, miseducation, mis-treatment, indifference, and last but not least, incredible stupidity.

That the sum of these characteristics could be possessed by all three doctors at the same time, in the same place, is nothing short of amazing. At any given time, one of them could have stepped forward and done the right thing. It was that simple and that easy.

However, I have learned from Phyllis that you can't just go around saying things about folks unless you have the evidence to back it up. So, let's take the doctor-foes and examine them one by one (no pun intended) to see if they have engaged in the weapons of body destruction listed above. We'll shuffle the deck of cards and see what our inspectors come up with.

First, the Joker-of-Clubs, Dr. Snyder. He's the Joker-of-Clubs because he was the first to knock me upside my head with the club he kept carefully concealed behind his back. He was the doctor that pressed the button and set the weapons of body destruction in motion. He used my body and trust abominably. It was such a simple thing for him to be responsible enough to at least learn all he could about UFEs *before* donating my body to an inexperienced interventional radiology group. No doubt, he would have done this if it were *his* testicles that were being embolized. And the sad thing is that Dr. Snyder did not know the radiology group was not experienced. He did not bother to inquire into their credentials. Some simple questions come to my mind and I am just a lowly layperson: How long have you been doing UFEs? How *many* UFEs have you performed? Will you be the doctor performing the UFE? What are the known adverse effects of UFE? Who will be responsible for the patient's follow up care? What is my expected involvement as the patient's gynecologist?

Even after it was clear that something had gone wrong with my UFE, it still did not occur to Dr. Snyder that it might be a good idea to read up on it. I guess he thought he had finished medical school and nobody was ever gonna make him do homework again! Was he really that lazy or was he just plain stupid? He obviously hadn't heard the saying that a man is himself, *plus* the books he reads. Where did he get his medical degree, anyway? From the University of Uterus R Us? To think it satisfied him to tell me that he did not know what to do but that he would keep trying to contact Dr. Rowley. The only solution he could come up with was to cut my uterus out of my body. No big deal. Aside from the fact that I had made it imminently clear, from day one, that I did not want a hysterectomy. He wanted to bury my uterus to hide his and Drs. Langford and Rowley's mistakes. As they say, if the doctor cures, the sun sees it; if he kills, the earth hides it. I guess I should be grateful that it was my uterus the earth is hiding instead of my body.

And let us not forget my six months of tortured suffering. If Dr. Snyder had done his homework, he would have known that what Dr. Rowley told him was just plain wrong. But since he did not know, he took everything Dr. Rowley said as true. Don't you think a red flag should have gone up at this point? Especially in light of the fact that he had initially been told, by Dr. Langford, that it was a simple 24-hour outpatient procedure where I would be fine after two days. Why would he believe Dr. Rowley was correct about six months, when Dr. Langford was clearly incorrect about two days? Did he even challenge Dr. Rowley on what he said and maybe pointed out to him that Dr. Langford had said something vastly different? I mean, help me out, am I expecting too much of three people who have aspired to the level of America's most respected? Is this not the essence of dumb, dumber, and dumbest? And as far as I'm concerned, they are all in a dead heat as to which one wins the dumbest prize. I think I'll give the dumbest prize to all of them; Dumbest, Mo'Dumbest, and The Dumbest.

Do you think it might have occurred to Dr. Snyder to call me and check up on me during the six month period? Well, no, because he still had not done any homework on UFEs so he had no way of knowing that I was walking around (when I could) with my uterus rotting inside me. Do you think he might have had some uneasiness about my condition since he had witnessed for himself that my uterus was larger, not smaller, when he examined me almost thirty days later? And that I was in tremendous pain and could not bear the touch of his examination? Duh! So even if I accept that he was not smart enough to figure it out, I would have happily settled for plain old concern and regard for a patient he mis-treated. Aren't doctors supposed to be our caregivers and healers? Well, this one lost sight of the goal line altogether, and went running wildly in the opposite direction.

And, still, there's more the inspectors have ferreted out on the Joker-of-Clubs. Dr. Snyder was the doctor that did not bother to call the hospital back on October 31, 2000 and, as a result, I was left laying on a gurney, without a blanket, in the hallway for over an hour. Determined not to die in the midst of this kind of indignity, I went home. Maybe the reason he could not call was because he was out somewhere trick-or-treating. After all it was Halloween. Let's see, what would be my guess as to what Halloween costume he was wearing. I got it! I can see it clearly. He has on a head-to-toe white jump suit, shaped in the form of a uterus, and pasted across the torso is a huge yellow circle trimmed in bright red, with a bright red line going diagonally through it. Around the circle are big black letters declaring, "Uterus Busters!"

And the most egregious conduct (well, maybe not, because there's still more) was when he "declined" to come to the hospital the next day on November 1, 2000 when I was so close to death that the Grim Reaper was already sharpening his knives to feast on my body. No sir, he was not coming anywhere near the mess he had helped to create with Drs. Langford and Rowley. Besides, he would not purposely put himself in a position where he might have to testify against the two villains that had hood-winked him. He knew I was dying, yet the doctor in him did not scream out for him to rush to the hospital to join the fight that was being waged to save my life. Incredible.

But, there's still more, and the inspectors themselves were appalled at this conduct. My insurance company refused to pay Dr. Snyder's bill because they said my treatment arose out of an experimental procedure, i.e., UFE. I tried to get the insurance company to pay the bill and they flat-footedly refused to pay the $1,545. Once Dr. Snyder realized the insurance company was not going to pay, he sicced his collection attack dogs on *me*. And little did I know that I would end up owing approximately $140,000 in medical bills from this doctor-foe's recommendation that he later ran and hid from.

Mind you, at the time, I was in the fight of my life just to stay alive from the destruction that had been caused by the negligence of the three doctor-foes. I was sick, weak, depressed, and unable to work. I spoke many times with the collection attack dog that called me repeatedly to get Dr. Snyder's money. I explained to her what had happened. I asked, "How can Dr. Snyder have the audacity to think I should pay him for nearly killing me? And the jury's still out on whether I'm going to make it! Can't he see the irony and injustice in this?" Well, no, he did not. He rendered medical service (never mind that it was service that nearly killed me) and, by golly, I was going to pay or else he would turn me over to a professional collection service that had *ferocious* collection attack dogs. And he did.

I begged and pleaded with his office not to allow this debt to be reported to the credit bureau. Since I was in the real estate investment business, negative credit ratings would be the kiss of death for me. It was clear that with Dr. Snyder I was doomed to die a thousand deaths. His powerful club was still knocking me upside my head. He reported the debt to the credit bureau so he was instrumental in effectively setting up road blocks to my livelihood.

So, have the inspectors and I convinced you that Dr. Snyder

was armed with the weapons of body destruction that I outlined above? I think we have.

Now, let's shuffle the deck of cards and see who comes out next. Ah, the Joker-of-Spades, Dr. Langford. When I talked with Dr. Langford, over the phone, he made sure that I would not come in for a face-to-face consultation. He did not want me to see the spade he was packing that might be useful if he needed to dig my grave. He knew Dr. Snyder had already sealed the deal for him so all he had to do was reiterate what he'd said to Dr. Snyder. He was slick as snot and he knew he had the advantage of being "the doctor." To a lowly little person like me, that was a powerful advantage because I had been raised to believe doctors were the pillars of our communities.

While Dr. Snyder hit me upside my head with his club, Dr. Langford slinked behind me, while I was not looking, and whacked me across my back with his sneaky-spade. He made me think he would be the doctor performing my UFE and even went to great lengths to make me believe this. He told me that he could do it that Friday, May 19, 2000, and he informed me the only way he could do it was if I would be willing to come to Hillside Hospital because he was scheduled to be there on that day. Now, as you might recall, I lived right around the corner from Butler Hospital. But, of course, I was willing to go way on the other side of town just to make sure Dr. Langford would perform my procedure. Of course I would want him to because my trusty Dr. Snyder had referred *him*.

Dr. Langford put me on hold, while he got his receptionist on the line, so she could make sure she scheduled the UFE under his name. And, oh yes, she had to make sure I gave her the insurance information to ensure that the interventional radiology group got paid their $7,500.

Apparently, somewhere along the way, Dr. Langford decided he did not want to do my UFE. Mayhap he planned it right from the beginning because the inspectors find it hard to believe that he could talk to me on a Tuesday, and not know where he was going to be scheduled for that Friday. Mayhap he got cold feet because he knew he had never performed a UFE before and decided he would shift the responsibility to a partner who had done *one*. In his mind, it must not have made a difference whether he or Dr. Rowley did my procedure because the money was still going into the radiology group pot. The only problem was that he neglected to tell me.

Did it not occur to him that I had the right to know if he was going to shift my body over to another doctor? Didn't he know he needed my authorization and consent before he could do this? Surely, he knew that this was not acceptable conduct in the medical community. All the experts that reviewed my case were revolted by the thought of a doctor doing this. And even Dr. Gunn, the expert that trained him, depicted it as "this sleight of hand switching of doctors." I've wrestled with this one because it just does not make sense to me. Maybe because he's a radiologist, he's not used to dealing with patients up close and personal. It would have been a good idea for him to take some bedside-manner classes before embarking into the field of UFEs where he would have to actually deal with patients face-to-face.

Dr. Langford never ever involved himself in any kind of follow up care. While he thought he had no responsibility as to my follow up care because he did not perform the procedure, he had no trouble turning me over to his partner because they were a radiology team. Well, what in the world happened to the team spirit when it came to my follow up care? Why could *he* not have returned Dr. Snyder's calls? He had slicked me into getting the UFE performed, so I guess he thought his job was done. He had performed his rain-maker function for the group.

So, you've got to agree that Dr. Langford's sneaky-spade turned out to be a powerful weapon of body destruction used against me.

Here comes our final shuffle of the cards. What have we here? If it isn't the Joker-of-Diamonds, Dr. Rowley. He is packing a bat as his weapon of body destruction because he is the one that went to bat for his radiology group. I'm sure it was his intent to hit a homerun but, instead, he nearly killed the specimen. He had performed one UFE so the radiology group must have been in awe of him and looked up to him with pride and expectation. And, indeed, he did swing his bat, but the only trouble is that instead of hitting a homerun, he hit me and knocked me out cold.

His follow up care for a patient that he performed a procedure on was equivalent to the worst case of abandonment in probably the whole history of medicine. I just refuse to believe that he is equaled anywhere. If he is, then we're all in a whole lot of trouble when it comes to medical care.

This doctor is the hardest for me because he is the one who butchered and maimed by body. And in my opinion he left me to die. As a matter of fact, all the doctor-foes did. When I think about how he put his hands on my body without my authorization and consent, my rage knows no bounds. When I think about how he carelessly told Dr. Snyder that it was normal for me to have symptoms for up to six months, I get weak with disbelief. When I think about how he never called to see how I was doing, I'm pure amazement. When I think about how Dr. Snyder tried to track him down for almost a month with no success, it makes me loathe him. When I think about how he put foreign objects in my body I had no knowledge of, it makes me despise him.

And there's something else the inspectors took note of Dr. Rowley and probably Dr. Langford too. A nurse from their office called me in July 2001, I guess to follow up on me and see how I was doing to see if I was someone they would want to report to the Fibroid Registry. I recall that I went into lengthy detail in telling her everything that happened to me up to that point. I'm sure I told her I was still having pain because I was. She appeared to be shocked by what I was telling her, especially the fact that I had not been pre-medicated with antibiotics. After getting an earfull of what I had to say, she promised to report everything I said to the doctors. Well, I want you to know I never heard back from the nurse or that office again.

Two things about this: 1) I was never ever reported to the Fibroid Registry by this interventional radiology group and if anybody should have been reported, it should have been me. Surely, the FDA would want to know about the horrendous adverse effects I was suffering. At least, I hope so; 2) Here was a clear opportunity for either Dr. Rowley, Dr. Langford, or *anybody in the radiology group* to have contacted me to. It was a last clear chance for *somebody* to do the right and decent thing. Instead, they swept me under the ole rug and tried to pretend I never happened.

That just about wraps up my case for my doctor-foes and their weapons of body destruction. I believe I've presented enough evidence to prove that they were packing powerful weapons in terms of nearly destroying my body, my family, and my finances.

The thing that bothers me the most is that I don't think the doctor-foes grasp the magnitude of what they have done to me and my family. In February 2003, my mother suffered a heart attack. I know that a lot of it had to do with all the stress she endured over nearly losing me on more than one occasion. She lived every day of my tortured existence for two years. I can still see my mother, on her hands and knees on the floor, cleaning up my vomit. She did this repeatedly over the course of two years. I know she still worries about me because of the last thing Dr. Olson said after my last surgery, "Kellee, expect the worse, and hope for the best."

I know my son was traumatized by what he had to witness during my long sojourn of illness. He was robbed of his mother at a most critical time in his life and I have always been front and center in his life. There's no telling what kind of fears are still harbored in his mind. He was dragged back and forth between Georgia and Ohio according to how my sickness was going.

Doctors, have you ever even given one thought as to how you

destroyed and broke down a life due to your incompetence and cavalier approach to medical treatment? Did you not know that you held my life in your hands and that if you did not take the care outlined in your Hippocratic Oath, that you might kill me? Remember, you're to "first do no harm." Do you care that you almost killed me? Your subsequent behavior has convinced me that you do not.

I have now decided what the dumbest line up should be: Dumbest, Dr. Langford; Mo' Dumbest, Dr. Rowley; and, The Dumbest, Dr. Snyder.

When Phyllis called in late October 2002, it was to tell me that the depositions of Drs. Langford and Rowley were scheduled for the middle of November. The law firm was still trying to get a date for the deposition of Dr. Snyder. His lawyer was being really slippery because we could not seem to get any dates that would work for him. I don't guess I would want my deposition taken if I was Dr. Snyder either. Who in their right mind would want to have to come and talk about how dumb they were?

We conducted my deposition and my mother's in mid-September. I was raked over the coals as opposing counsel dug into every nook and cranny of my life. I was so worried about my mother having to go through this ordeal and I sat in the room with her while her deposition was being taken.

I felt my throat tighten up when the opposing counsel, Mr. Marlowe, asked my mother, "Is there any family history of depression?"

"No," she answered.

He asked, "As a child, did she ever require any kind of psychiatric or psychological—"

"No," she said, "This was one of the happiest people in the world at the end of this table until this all happened. We did so many things together and just had fun all the time."

I felt like crying when I heard this exchange but I would never allow my enemies to see me cry. Sadly, I could not remember the last time we had fun. I was too busy being afraid of when the next shoe was going to drop. I was better now in the sense that I refused to give up on any of this without a fight.

When I talked to Phyllis, I told her I wanted to be present at all the doctors' depositions. Wild horses could not have kept me away. I had never seen Drs. Langford and Rowley and there was no way I was going to miss the opportunity to get an up close look at the two doctors who had such a crucial part in the destruction of my life. I wanted to face my demons. I wanted to look them straight in the face if they lied. Phyllis and Joseph had counseled me thoroughly on how I was to not, in any way, show any emotion during the depositions. They warned me that I might get angry at some of the things the doctors said but I would have to keep tight control of my emotions.

The day arrived for the depositions. The first to be deposed was Dr. Langford who raised his right hand and swore to tell the truth. The same right hand he used to hold the phone receiver while conducting his deception against me.

I watched with admiration as Phyllis conducted the deposition. I watched and listened intently to every response. After all, this was a part of my life that was in the dark that was now coming to the light. She was persistent in her questioning and made it very difficult for them to slither out of answering. My ears really perked up when it got to the part that had to do with his knowledge about UFEs.

"Doctor," Phyllis asked, "did you ever teach a seminar on uterine fibroid embolization?

"Yes, I did," he answered.

"And when did you do that?"

"I gave a lecture to the Ob/Gyn department meeting at Butler Hospital, I'm not sure exactly what time period but it would probably have been 1999 or 2000 just to give them an overview of the procedure. There had been a lot of requests generated in general by women who had either seen articles in the newspaper or on the television or on the Internet and they were bringing a lot of their concerns and questions to the gynecologist and there was not a lot of information yet for the gynecologists to draw on. So they wanted some background on the procedure and what the process was and some of the different aspects of it."

"Now, at the time that you gave this lecture, Doctor, had you yourself performed any uterine fibroid embolizations?"

My ears *really* perked up.

"No, I had not done fibroid embolization. I had done uterine artery embolization for bleeding but not fibroid embolization," he answered.

Well, doesn't that beat all? He was giving lectures on something he had not even done?

My mouth may be silent but my mind is working like a Jumbo-Jet that has taken off. I'm not going to pass up this opportunity to carry on a mental dialogue with Dumbest.

Now they are talking about when Dr. Gunn came and gave a lecture before the radiology group. I honed in again.

"Do you recall when Dr. Gunn was here giving this lecture, Doctor?" Phyllis asked.

"I don't," he answered. "I think it was in the fall of 1999, it might have been the winter but I'm not sure."

"And did Dr. Gunn come as a result of a specific request by your radiology group or was it something that was scheduled by the Society of Interventional Radiologists?"

"No, our radiology group and our interventional radiology subsection requested him to come down and paid for him to come down and give a lecture to the Gyn physicians as well as to us interventional radiologists both formally and informally."

Sounds like a whole cash crop had sprung up around UFEs. I'll bet this will make doctors a lot of money if they can get enough bodies donated to experiment on. Every interventional radiologist should be lucky enough to have a Dr. Snyder in their back pocket.

"Could you go into a bit more detail as to the informal training that he gave to the radiologists at this particular time?" Phyllis asked.

"Well, I don't remember specifics but in general when people tell you about the procedure they tell you how they did it, what their technique is, what their indications are for the procedure, what their expectations are for success or for failure and for complications and that's what he had done with us," Dr. Langford answered.

They moved to another topic of interest to me.

"Doctor, when was the first time you performed a uterine fibroid embolization procedure?" Phyllis asked.

"I don't know the exact date but it was sometime in mid 2000, mid to late 2000," he answered.

"In mid 2000, did you exercise the use of coils in this procedure?"

"I never use coils in a uterine artery embolization for fibroids, although people were doing it at that time, I just elect not to. People were doing both."

"Why did you elect not to use them?"

"At that time the teaching was that the uterine artery should be completely embolized and coils will completely embolize the vessel."

Well, it sure completely embolized my vessel! Yes sir, it completely shut down all the blood flow to my uterus and damn near the rest of my body. That's why I ended up with a dead carcass of a uterus inside me. And "at that time" bothers me. Sounds like the only part you were sure of was the script you used to bait me in.

I'm really getting into my mental commentary.

"A coil is an extra step and I elected not to perform the extra step," Dr. Langford was saying. "There was discussion both formally and informally at that time that if you didn't completely embolize the uterine artery that you would have an incomplete embolization and that you would have a lesser chance of success…"

Here goes that "at that time" again! I think what that means is "we know better now." How do they know better? At my expense, of course.

"…a poorer response to the procedure, more likelihood that

the symptoms would continue. And so I just elected to embolize it completely with the particles alone. It was just easier I guess is probably the bottom line."

Am I hearing this correctly? There was no uniform way for doctors to perform UFEs? It was just up for grabs and doctors could do it anyway they thought they wanted to do it? They could just freely practice on women without knowing for sure which was the best method? Some use coils and some don't? What kind of practice of medicine is this? Why hadn't the issue of whether or not to use coils been thoroughly researched before the first uterine fibroid embolization was marketed to the general public?

Oh, I get it. Women in the general public are the test market, only the doctors get to make $7,500 per procedure while they practice. After all, the only thing at stake is a little ole insignificant uterus. That's no big deal. We'll just cut it out if it starts acting up and causing us any trouble. And the only reason Dr. Langford didn't use coils was because it was easier, i.e., less trouble for him to be bothered with? Like how he didn't want to be bothered with me once he had slicked me into getting the procedure. Interesting.

Now they are talking about the Fibroid Registry and from what I am hearing, it does not appear he knew much about that either. *Is this for real?*

"Doctor, you've already stated that you are a UAE Fibroid Registry participating physician. Would you explain what the UAE Fibroid Registry is?" Phyllis asked.

"I think I can explain, too, in general, I'm not involved in the management of it or in the process of doing it, we have a nurse practitioner who is helping us with that but that's through the Society of Interventional Radiology to register patients that are having fibroids for research. And I don't know where our—I don't know where we stand on that as far as if we're active in it or if we're still making application process or what. I can just tell you that I know we're involved in the discussions with the Society of being on the Registry and I believe we're on the Registry but I'm not sure."

"But on your website you do hold yourself out as being a Fibroid Registry participating physician."

"Right, because I believe we are."

You believe? You don't know?

"Do you know what the requirements are for you becoming a participating physician under the Fibroid Registry?" she asked.

"I don't know any of the specific requirements, no," he answered.

Dumbest times one.

"How many UFEs have you performed to date?" Phyllis asked.

"I think I've performed somewhere around eight but I'm not sure of the exact number," he said.

What! You don't know the exact number of your UFE patients? I see now. They're in the Registry of Cadavers. Watch out doc, you're not keeping up with the notches on your belt.

"You wouldn't know whether or not you reported any complications to the Fibroid Registry?"

"No."

"Did you have any training in the gynecologic aspects of the UFE procedure?"

"The only gynecologic training I would have had would have been in medical school and that did not relate to uterine fibroid embolization, as that was not a procedure at that time."

Yikes! No training in gynecology and you guys had the nerve to hold yourselves out as experts in uterine fibroid embolization? Clueless about the uterus. Dumbest times two.

Now Phyllis is honing in on the experimental, A.K.A., investigational status of UFE. This is really getting good and juicy.

"Now, let's distinguish between uterine artery embolization and uterine fibroid embolization. I am aware that uterine artery embolization has been around for a long time. But uterine fibroid embolization is something that is fairly new. Isn't that correct?" she asked.

171

"That's correct."

"Now, as a result of that would it not be referred to as an investigational procedure at this point?"

"I don't know how it's referred to. That could very well be true, I don't know."

"Do you know, Doctor, what they mean when they say investigational?"

"When the term is used?" he asked. "No, I'm not sure of the exact legal implication of that. Obviously I can understand the general implications of what being investigational means, it means it's being investigated as to how successful the procedure is and...but I don't know who would deem that."

Bully for you! You're finally getting on the right track with a little prodding.

Phyllis is relentless and is not backing off.

"Do you think perhaps that is the reason the Fibroid Registry has been set up?" she asked.

"It's a good possibility," Dr. Langford answered.

Amazing. Are they just giving away medical degrees these days? Dumbest times three.

Phyllis is switching tactics.

"Do you know the percentage of women that end up having a hysterectomy after a UFE procedure?" she asked.

"I don't know the exact percentage, I know relative percentages are low but that has evolved a bit because the procedures been new," he answered.

Oh! Dumbest. This is not a shining moment for you!

As it turns out, he doesn't know much about the issue of fertility either.

"Doctor, in terms of the patients that you performed UFEs on in 2000, do you recall if any of them were interested in preserving their fertility?" Phyllis asked.

"No, I don't recall. Though, in general almost every patient we get is interested in preserving their uterus and oftentimes that's for potential for fertility in the future. But I don't—I have no—I don't know the specifics of any of the patients," he answered.

"Maybe I should be more specific with it. Were any of your patients that you performed the procedure on in 2000 interested in having children?" she asked.

"I don't remember."

Umph-umph-umph!

"For 2001?"

"I don't remember that either."

Umph-umph-umph!

"And for 2002?"

"Same thing."

Unbelievable! What's next? Drive-thru UFEs? Dumbest times four.

My head is spinning. I would not have missed this for the entire world. It's like watching a not-so-well-put-together soap opera. Now they are getting into who would be the best candidate for UFEs. This should really be enlightening. Especially since they don't know anything about the patients and it's obviously not a requirement.

"Who would be a good candidate for UFE?" Phyllis asked.

"Maybe from general to specific, in general the patient that's good for fibroid embolization has symptoms and they're usually bleeding or pressure symptoms from the fibroids. If there's no symptoms then there's no reason to do the procedure," he said.

Well, doctor, as you might recall I didn't have any symptoms so what was the reason to do the procedure on me? But then again, how would you have known I did not have symptoms since you're not required to know anything about the patient or the procedure. Maybe your motivation was $7,500.

"The second thing that's uniform and universal as best I can tell is that they want to maintain their uterus and there can be different reasons for that, there can be fertility reasons, there could be the desire not to have an incision on their abdomen..."

But, doctor! I ended up with an ugly scar on my abdomen from an incision. And it's so ugly because they had to go in and cut me open twice in the same place. For your information, this was due to my UFE. Obviously, my vanity wasn't an issue.

"...there could be the desire to hopefully return to work within one to two weeks as opposed to six weeks."

Hopefully? Well you blew it on that one! It's been over two years since my UFE and I'm still not able to hit the floor and give twenty.

"I think in general those are the two main things that we have to get past. If there's not symptoms and there's not a desire to maintain the uterus, then we probably don't need to go a whole lot further than that," he said.

I'm too through!

On the next issue Dumbest really not-shines.

"In 2000 what was your standard protocol when you got a UFE patient?" Phyllis asked.

"The initial contact is by telephone. At that point the patient's really given the option if they would like to discuss more they could come in and see us. And, like I said, in 2000 we had a procedure where we'd have them come to the hospital and we would find a private room somewhere in the radiology department to have a more in-depth discussion with the patient. Or at that point if they felt comfortable by the discussion by telephone they could be scheduled for the procedure at that point," he said.

Or, as in my case, you were already sent to the torture chamber by your gynecologist.

"So in 2000 you didn't feel that it was absolutely necessary to have a face-to-face consultation with the patient prior to performing a UFE?" she asked.

"No, I wouldn't say that's true, we definitely have a face-to-face conversation but that can happen just before the procedure when the patient has already made the decision to have it, or it could happen at a separate time days before. That option was given to the patient," he said.

Well now doc, I beg to differ with you on this point. It was not a matter of an option with me. You told me I didn't need to come in for a face-to-face consultation because it was just a simple 24-hour outpatient procedure. Besides, an advanced meeting would have prevented an effective bait and switch.

"What I said was face-to-face *consultation*," she said.

"That's correct," he replied.

"And what I mean by that, that's more to me than a conversation. It's where just like you're saying, a patient would want to know all the information and likewise you would want to know information about the patient during this consultation. Isn't that correct?" she asked.

"No, I don't think that's correct. They were given a potential to either have a face-to-face if you want to call it a consultation either a separate time or at the time just before their procedure when they were already at the hospital," he said.

Right. Like when they've already been shot up with a tranquilizer and don't know what the hell is going on or could give a shit. You'd better watch it, Doc, you're approaching Dumbest times five.

"So in 2000 you didn't feel it was mandatory to have a face-to-face consultation with you?" Phyllis persisted.

"That's not what I'm saying. I'm saying they have a face-to-face consultation either before the procedure in terms of a day or a week or a month, or that same day," he said.

Umph- umph-umph!

And it gets worse.

"Was it your practice in 2000 to perform any kind of physical examination of the patient prior to the UFE procedure?" Phyllis asked.

"No, in general we did not perform a physical examination just because of the office constraints, we were talking to people, not doing a physical examination. A physical examination generally would happen on the day of the procedure anyway," he said.

Oh, my God! That's kinda like closing the gate after the horses have escaped, isn't it? Isn't the physical examination for the purpose of telling you whether the patient should even have a UFE? But if she's already scheduled for it before the physical examination, what's the point? Or maybe, the bed in the hall didn't have stirrups attached. No doubt about it, this is Dumbest times five!

"How did you and Dr. Snyder come to discuss Kellee Kendell in reference to a uterine fibroid embolization?" she asked

This should be really good. I'd better pay really close attention.

"Again with the help of the materials from this case I received a phone call from Dr. Snyder about uterine fibroid embolization and that he had a patient that he thought was a candidate for uterine fibroid embolization," he answered.

"Do you dispute that that conversation took place, doctor?" Phyllis asked.

"I don't recall it." he answered.

Oh no! You mean to tell me I was the first fish he hooked and he remembers nothing about how he snagged me? I can understand people forgetting about the one that got away. But the first big fish you catch you always remember. I'm disappointed.

"You don't recall any of the specifics of the conversation?" she asked.

"I don't recall the specifics of the conversation," he answered.

How convenient not to recall. Now, I'm no lawyer but I'm very familiar with the "I don't recall" strategy. It gets you off the hook so nobody can nab you for what you really do recall. Do you recall your generous donation of my body to Dr. Rowley?

Phyllis persisted.

"And the only reason you remember anything is because of the written materials that you've reviewed as a result of this case?" she said.

"That's correct," he answered.

"Did you tell Dr. Snyder that you had never performed a UFE procedure?"

"I don't recall."

"Have you and Westside Radiology received any more referrals for UFE from Dr. Snyder?"

"I don't know."

You're doing really well on the know-nothing strategy doc. You make your lawyers proud.

"Now, in answers to our interrogatories you stated you had a conversation with Ms. Kendell prior to her procedure; is that correct?" Phyllis asked.

"Again, I don't have recollection of that but that's what's in the materials and that sounds reasonable as to what would have happened," he answered.

My, my, my. He specifically stated in his interrogatories what our conversation was but here in person, his recollection is based on the materials in the case file? Maybe his recollection is affected because I'm sitting glaring at him with my amazing good looks and sparkling personality.

"No," Phyllis persisted, "this was in your answers to our interrogatories. We specifically asked you in the interrogatories whether or not you had a conversation with Ms. Kendell. And your answer was yes, that you had."

Mr. Marlowe jumped in to his client's defense and said, "Objection, that's argumentative."

Now, help me out. I'm confused. Phyllis is arguing with the doc just because she wants to know why he specifically stated in his interrogatories that he had a conversation with me and now he's saying he only wrote that because of what was in the file? Excuse me, but there was no file. And if this is the case, how can that be a proper answer? Wouldn't his correct answer to the interrogatory be "I don't recall?"

"So my question is do you recall that you answered in your interrogatory that you had a conversation with Ms. Kendell?" Phyllis asked, again.

"I don't recall what I answered in the interrogatory if that's what you're asking."

Now that sounds reasonable because you probably didn't answer the interrogatories, your lawyers did. Just like you didn't do the procedure. Your partner did.

"Doctor, do you specifically recall discussing the complications with Kellee Kendell?" she asked.

"No I don't directly recall that," he answered.

"And you also stated in your interrogatories that you discussed the risks of the procedure with Ms. Kendell, and we've already talked about the risks earlier on in the deposition. Do you have any specific recollection of having discussed the risks with Ms. Kendell?"

"No."

"You state in your answers to our interrogatories that you discussed the effect of UFE on fertility with Ms. Kendell. Do you have specific recollection of discussing the effect on fertility that UFE might have?"

"No."

"You also state in your answers to our interrogatories that you discussed the advantages and disadvantages of the UFE procedure. Do you have specific recollection of what advantages and disadvantages you discussed with Ms. Kendell?"

"No."

Phyllis! You're being ruthless. I love it! You go girl!

"You state in your answers to our interrogatories that there were other things you discussed with Ms. Kendell. What were the other things you discussed with Ms. Kendell?"

"I don't have any specific recollection of any other things."

"During your conversation with Ms. Kendell did you ever tell her you had never performed a UFE procedure?"

"I don't recall."

Well, I recall. You didn't. If you had, I would have run like a scared rabbit does from the sudden glare of oncoming headlights.

"You state in your answers to our interrogatories that Ms. Kendell was responsible for her decision to ignore the advice of her doctors. What was the advice of her doctors that Ms. Kendell decided to ignore?"

Mr. Marlowe spoke up and said, "Object to the form."

"I'm not…I don't understand the question. I'm not sure what advice that is," Dr. Langford said.

Just like you didn't understand the procedure. I knew it was coming. Dumbest times six.

"Or what your lawyer said," Mr. Marlowe piped in. "Since the lawyers draft the responses commonly, or at least some of the language within them."

Well now, the cat's out of the bag. I was right and I feel vindicated. The lawyers drafted the answers to the interrogatories. My only question is, if the lawyers drafted the answers, why didn't they sign the interrogatories? Umph-umph-umph!

As Mark Twain so aptly put it, "Let's put a curtain of charity over the rest of this scene!"

Chapter Ten

Mo Demons!

Well, I thought I would be finished facing my demons in the last chapter but there was so much to record that I had to carry it over into another chapter. I apologize for having to drag you through another chapter but there are mo' demons I think you need to know about. I have to say I was appalled at what I learned as a result of Dr. Langford's deposition. If there ever was a time that Murphy's Law was firmly entrenched, I think you have to agree it was operating full-time in my case.

Can you believe that the radiology group would start culling the field for prospective UFE patients *before* they even set up shop? I mean, they didn't even have an office where they could see patients! I can see it now. An examination table with stirrups, facing the handicapped section of the parking lot. And Dr. Langford had the audacity to teach a seminar on UFEs to the gynecologists and he had never performed even one UFE! Now, I know Dr. Langford is going to come after me with the explanation, "but I have done numerous uterine artery embolizations (UAEs) so I have a plethora of experience in the embolization of the uterine arteries. So I *am* an expert at performing this procedure."

The only trouble is that when radiologists did UAEs it was for women who were hemorrhaging. That's big-time different than doing the procedure for uterine fibroids. So, wouldn't it be just plain common sense to know that if you're doing embolization for fibroids instead of for hemorrhaging, it just might have a different effect on the uterus? And, by the way, this is why UFE snuck so cleverly through the FDA because, indeed, the doctors could show that embolization was not a new procedure. We've been doing it for over twenty years guys! It's only the *use* for the procedure that's different and that's no big deal. We're experts at this because we have done numerous UAEs, i.e., we don't have to do any additional training for UFEs and we already know all we need to know about the uterus.

Now that is scary. Wouldn't performing embolization for fibroids require at least a modicum of understanding about the functioning of the female reproductive organs? It never occurred to these bozos, and apparently the teaching radiologists, that it should be a mandatory requirement that interventional radiologists get some basic training in the aspect of gynecology that would pertain to uterine *fibroid* embolization. Or, at the very least, have a clear plan as to how they could work in collaboration with the gynecologists so the safest medical care could be rendered to the patient.

I was caught in a maelstrom that just kept getting worse and worse. And it kept getting worse due to the unbelievable ignorance and stupidity of the doctor-foes. The gynecologist didn't know diddly-squat about the UFE and the interventional radiologists didn't know diddly-squat about gynecologic issues. And the two disciplines failed to communicate effectively with each other or have a plan in the beginning about how this would work. Apparently, the only plan the interventional radiologists had was to make $7,500 per procedure. I'm convinced that this is what put the stars in their eyes.

All they had to do was take one more step: educate

themselves about gynecologic issues or clearly coordinate a path to work closely with the gynecologists. It seems to me that the first thing that would come out of the instructor's mouths would be, "Fellas you've got to understand gynecologic issues, regarding fibroids, *before* you embark on this course." Women can be very complicated. Even I know that.

The really big shock for me was to learn that there is no general consensus on how the uterine fibroid embolization is to be performed. Some doctors use coils along with the polyvinyl alcohol particles and some doctors do not. It seems to me that very little has been done to get complete clarification on this point. And even as a layperson, I can see that the docs need to really agree on this. I surely know that in my case, coils were used, and, in my case, my uterus died from the use of the polyvinyl alcohol particles in conjunction with the coils. The addition of the coils completely shut off the blood supply to my uterus. Doesn't what is the safest and best method for performing UFEs just scream, MORE RESEARCH!?

The only reason Dr. Langford chooses not to use the coils is because it's just one more step he doesn't want to deal with. I'd feel a lot better if he said he did it because he thought it was more effective and safer than using the coils. And this is probably what he really thinks, but, he can't say that because then he would be saying that he did not agree with the way his partner, Dr. Rowley, did it. What's really scary about this is, if they don't have a consensus within their own group for performing UFEs, what else must be going on in interventional radiology cyberspace? Be afraid, be very afraid.

I could go on and on with this because it seems like it's never-ending. However, I need to move on and tell you about what happened with Dr. Rowley's deposition the next day. I think you'll find Mo' Dumbest to be just as incompetent and unknowledgeable as his partner, Dumbest.

Phyllis was her usual feisty self and I must say, I enjoyed watching her rake Dr. Rowley over the coals. Of course, I gave my usual mental commentary which I think you'll find as interesting and as amusing as yesterday with Dr. Langford. I mean, I've had to develop a sense of humor in all this because, if I had not, I could have easily embarked on a nervous breakdown. Many times I had to laugh to keep from crying. Many times.

After intently witnessing yesterday's deposition, I left the building feeling immensely grateful to have escaped with my life. It was nothing short of a miracle, considering I was in the hands of three incompetent doctors.

Dr. Rowley, while being sworn in by the court reporter, raised his right hand and swore to tell the truth. I could not help but look at that hand and realize this was the same hand that was used to mutilate and maim me.

We were not far into his deposition before I clearly saw why Dr. Rowley had earned Mo' Dumbest in the dumbest line up.

"How did you come to decide to incorporate the performance of uterine fibroid embolizations into your practice?" Phyllis asked.

"The then-president of the practice, who is also an interventional radiologist in our group, had been to a recent meeting where this was discussed in detail and we invited an expert to come give a talk. And then because, you know, the procedure involves procedures that were techniques that we already were well aware of and well versed in doing, you know, we proceeded to offer the procedure as an alternative," Dr. Rowley answered.

I don't know about the "well versed" part, doc. The proof is in the pudding and I'm pretty botched up. Is that the alternative you're talking about?

I know, I've started really early with the mental dialogue, but I can't help myself. Besides, you want to hear from me, don't you? After all, this is the doctor-foe that butchered and maimed me which resulted in an ugly scar tattooed on my abdomen for the rest of my life. The only thing that could be worse would be his picture tattooed on my abdomen.

"Doctor, when you were talking about the lecture that you attended that was kind of hosted by Dr. Thomas King, do you recall who was in charge of that lecture, who was giving the lecture that year?" she asked.

"Dr. Gunn," he answered.

"And what was the content of that particular lecture?"

"I was not present at that lecture. I understand that he gave a talk on uterine fibroid embolization."

You didn't even go to the lecture?

"Then I assume that someone told you about the lecture?" she asked.

"Yes," he said.

"As a result of that information, that's when you decided that you wanted to be involved in UFEs?'

"As a group we made that decision, yes."

Made the decision to what? Cash in on the UFE cash cow?

Oh, here we go, Phyllis is getting to the bottom of this now.

"When you say as a group, was there a meeting of the doctors at Westside Radiology?"

"It may have been an informal meeting, but it was—it may not have been a called meeting, but you know, we as a group decided that, yes."

I guess it's not necessary to call a meeting to discuss $7,500 per procedure. Everybody would agree on this no-brainer, present or not present. Maybe they should have used the dimple chad system.

"Dr. Rowley, how many UFE procedures have you performed?"

"I have performed approximately ten."

"And you performed your first one in March 2000?"

"Yes, ma'am."

"Doctor can you tell me why you decided to use coils in this particular procedure?"

I really want to hear this. I'm glad Phyllis is asking why he decided to use coils in my procedure instead of a hammer, nuts, and bolts.

"Coils at that time were an option to what was termed complete embolization."

Here we go with the "at that time" again. Remember, this really means "we know better now."

"So do you believe the embolization could not have been completed without the use of coils?"

"I can't answer that without, you know, kind of knowing that, you know—you know, theoretically, yes, it could have been completed with more and more of the same material that we are using."

"Now, do you still use coils in your UFE procedures?"

"No."

"When did you stop using them?"

"I stopped using them somewhere in the summer of 2000 or so."

"Would that have been after Kellee Kendell's procedure?"

"Yes."

I knew it! All along I've been saying I was used as a guinea pig. I'm vindicated, once again.

It gets better.

"And why did you decide to stop using the coils, Doctor?"

"It was at that time that I believe that more of the teaching and the literature began to support the fact that we might need to move more toward, you know, an incomplete embolization to some extent or a less of an embolization that was being performed previously."

What does that mean? Allowing the patient to keep her life and only lose her uterus? I've had enough of this. I've learned all I need to know on this issue—I was used like a cadaver, period.

Listen up, it's starting to get even more enlightening.

"Now, doctor, are some of the journals that you read, are they journals that are written by Ob/Gyns?"

"I don't review the Ob/Gyn literature. I review the radiology literature."

Mo' Dumbest times one.

"Did you take any CME courses that may have been taught by Ob/Gyns that had to do with uterine fibroid embolizations?"

"I don't believe so, no."

The next topic is really good, and Mo' Dumbest doesn't shine any brighter than Dumbest.

"Now, you state in your answers to interrogatories that you participate in reporting cases to the uterine Fibroid Registry?" Phyllis asked.

"Yes," he answered.

"How many cases have you reported to the Registry?"

"I honestly don't know."

Oh, come on doc! You've only done ten UFEs. This should have been a no-brainer. But we have to consider who's being asked the question.

"Is uterine fibroid embolization considered an investigational procedure?" she said.

"Define investigational," he said.

Oh my God Mo' Dumbest! Aren't you the doctor?

"I was hoping you could define that for me." Phyllis said

That's right Phyllis, make him earn that M.D. behind his name.

"It is investigational only in the sense that it is not known at this point what the optimal embolization procedure entails and what the long-term outcomes are to fibroid embolization and along those lines."

Dead-on-balls-accurate Mo' Dumbest! But, wait a minute. It's investigational only in the sense that it is not known at this point what the optimal embolization procedure entails? Isn't that big-time important? That's why some of you guys are using coils and some of you are not because you don't have the research to tell you what the hell to do. You're making it up as you go along at the expense of women. This is ticking me off Mo' Dumbest. My botched up UFE gave you some big clues on what the long-term outcomes could be and you didn't bother to report it to the Fibroid Registry. The pitiful thing is, you don't realize the significance of what you just said. Mo' Dumbest times two.

Phyllis is being relentless again.

"So along those lines it would be considered investigational at this stage?" she persisted.

"Yes," he said.

Umph-umph-umph!

"Is uterine fibroid embolization considered experimental?"

"I don't believe so, no."

"When you say you don't believe so, do you have some question about that?"

"No."

"So your answer would be it's not experimental?"

"Yes."

I beg to differ with you. You guys haven't figured out whether to use coils or not and some of you are still using them. You haven't figured out the long term outcomes to UFE over a period of at least ten years, either. Wasn't what you did to my body an experiment, i.e., using me like you might a cadaver? Everything that could have gone wrong did go wrong. Did you learn anything from my experiment? But, I know, I know. Investigational sounds a lot less frightening. You guys sure know how to play on words and use it to your advantage.

I'd better pay attention. Phyllis is really testing his intelligence now.

"Doctor, do you know the percentage of women that end up having hysterectomies after they have had a UFE?" she asked.

"The—I don't know the specific number but it's extremely low," he said.

"How do you know that it's extremely low?"

"It's—I would only venture a guess as to the exact number, but it's—in a way it depends on what the reason for the hysterectomy, you know, was performed after a UFE."

Maybe you can depend on finding out the reason when the autopsy report comes in. You don't know the answer to this question and you're trying to wing it. I can help you out on some of this Mo' Dumbest. In my case, I had to have a hysterectomy because you plugged my uterine arteries up so tight that you cut off all the blood supply to my uterus.

It's kinda like what happens when you tie a rubber band around your finger. Only, the rubber band couldn't be taken off my uterus so it turned black and rotted inside me slowly infecting my other organs for almost six months.

Phyllis is switching topics.

"Can you tell us, Doctor, whether or not women who are interested in having children would be considered appropriate candidates for participation in the UAE Fibroid Registry?" she asked.

"Only after counseling that the procedure does not guarantee fertility. And if that were their primary concern was to maintain their fertility, I would recommend them not to have the procedure done," he said.

Obviously scripted. That wasn't the question Mo' Dumbest.

"I do appreciate that answer, Doctor, but specifically I was asking as it relates to UAE and the Fibroid Registry. Are patients who are interested in having children considered appropriate candidates for this study?"

"I don't know."

Umph-umph-umph!

Now we're moving into another area.

"Do you work in collaboration with the referring physician if you go forward with the UFE?" she asked.

"In the sense that we keep them apprised if the patient has undergone, what things have gone on with the procedure and how the patient is doing, to the best of our knowledge," he said.

Oh, really?

"And how do you keep the referring physician apprised?"

"Are we talking current or past?" he asked

"I would like for you to tell me in 2000 and current," she said.

"In the year 2000 we would—if—you know, it might be a follow-up call, it might be a casual conversation in the hallway. There was nothing formal. There were no, to my knowledge, I don't think we were sending letters out at that time.

A casual conversation in the hallway? You bet there was nothing formal. You just left me to die. I can tell you for sure, you weren't sending out letters in 2000, you weren't even making an appearance. You weren't even sending out phone calls. That's why I labeled you the phantom doctor.

Now Phyllis is getting to the real nitty-gritty.

"After the consultations that you have with these patients, do you do a physical examination?" she asked.

"Yes, we do now," he said.

"When you say yes, we do now, this was not true in 2000?"

"In 2000 we would do that physical exam once the patient came to the hospital. Because at that time, in 2000, we did not have an exam room available to us."

"And there was no where in the hospital in 2000 that you could have performed a physical exam and a consultation prior to the UFE procedure?"

"There was, unfortunately, there was just no room available where we could do that sort of thing."

That sort of "thing"? And unfortunately your radiology group couldn't wait until you did have office space to have face-to-face consultations and physical examinations. Not being set up properly was not going to stop you from making $7,500 per procedure.

Listen to this one.

"Doctor, do you think it's important to have a face-to-face consultation with the patient prior to performing the UFE procedure?" Phyllis asked.

"All patients are seen face-to face prior to the procedure, whether it be just before, so in a sense there is a face-to-face prior to every procedure. But, I don't think it's important that you see the patient face-to-face prior to arranging to have the procedure done." Dr. Rowley answered.

That's right. All you need is a groin-to-face session so you can collect your $7,500. And you don't want to alert the patient to all the risks of UFE and scare them off. Mo' Dumbest times two.

"So what you're saying then, Doctor, is if a patient calls up and says I just want to learn more about the UFE procedure and learn more about the doctors before I have the procedure done, you would not consider it important to bring that patient in to have a consultation with you?"

"No."

Umph-umph-umph!

"Now when you say the interventional suite there at the hospital, was it set up like an office?"

"No, it's a procedure room."

"Just a procedure room?"

"Yes."

"With a phone?"

"Yes."

So how could you have done a physical exam and consultation with me doc?

Now they're entering into an entirely different subject matter. I'm really interested in this.

"When did you first see Kellee Kendell, Dr. Rowley, face-to-face?" Phyllis asked.

"I first met Ms. Kendell in the hallway outside the angio suite prior to her being brought into the room for the procedure," he answered.

As I've pointed out before, by this time I was all shot up with tranquilizer and didn't know what the hell was going on and could give a shit.

"When you say out in the hallway, was she on a gurney or was she sitting up in a chair?"

"She was on a gurney."

"And did she have an IV going at that time?"

"Yes."

See? I told you!

"And this was out in the hallway because there was no room available at that time where you could have taken her for a consultation?"

"Yes."

Umph-umph-umph!

"And there was no room available where you could have taken her specifically for a physical examination either?"

"True."

I always knew it! You copied exactly what the nurse wrote when I first came to the hospital for my UFE and wrote it on the doctor physical exam page, then signed your name to it. That way, it would make it look like you gave me a physical exam. But now you admit there was no place to give me a physical exam or the equipment to do it with. Clearly, Mo' Dumbest times three.

But Phyllis is still hot on his heels.

"Was there anyone else present when you first saw her in the hallway on the gurney?"

"I don't recall."

"What did you do, what was the first thing you did when you saw her?"

"I greeted her and asked her if she had any further questions about the procedure. I always give a little brief synopsis of what the procedure entails just so if there are any last minute questions or concerns, and you know, and answer those questions."

But, Mo' Dumbest, I was shot full of my happy-shot by this time! That's why I don't remember ever seeing you or remembering anything about the procedure. I do remember when the nurse gave me the shot and that was before they took me over to the radiology suite. I don't care what the medical records say. The radiology suite was in another location in the hospital from where I was when I first came to the hospital. I know the nurse didn't follow me over to the radiology suite, with happy shot in hand, waiting for you to talk to me while I was still in my right mind. No, I don't think anyone would believe it happened that way. You'd better watch it, you're stacking up your Mo' Dumbest points really fast. Mo' Dumbest times four.

"Now, as you were talking with Ms. Kendell out in the hallway, I'm trying to get a feel for what kind of hallway this is, are there other people walking by up and down the hallway, or do you have privacy there or no?" Phyllis was asking.

Oh, Phyllis! You're moving in for the kill now! You get 'em girl!

"There are people that—I mean, it's a hallway that is an access to different departments in the hospital, so I mean, people do occasionally walk by."

Umph-umph-umph!

'Was that a kind of busy day that day where people might have been walking by?"

That's right Phyllis, don't let him slither off the hook!

"They may have, yes."

Bingo!

Well, Phyllis wore him out so much that he said he needed a break. But when they went back on the record, it was clear she had sharpened her knives even more.

"Doctor how long does it normally take to perform the UFE procedure?" she asked.

"Typically, from the time that the artery is accessed until the procedure is completely done, can vary any where from an hour and a half to two to three hours. It just varies on the arterial anatomy and how difficult it is to gain access to it." he said.

You must have forgotten to discuss this point with Dumbest and The Dumbest. They told me the procedure would only take thirty to forty-five minutes. That's a big difference from what you're saying, isn't it? Is this your way of justifying the $7,500 fee?

"Do you recall how long it took to do Kellee's?"

"I don't recall."

Watch this. This is really good stuff.

"Doctor, I would like to direct your attention to pages 27 and 28 of Plaintiff's Exhibit Number Five and ask that you identify that page for me please?"

"This is the procedure consent form."

"What is the procedure or the title on that page for the procedure?"

"The procedure is embolization of intrauterine fibroids."

"Is that what it states at the top of the page?"

"Very top?" he asked.

"Yes," she said.

"Consent for diagnostic procedure involving contrast media," he answered.

That's right Phyllis, make him tell it like it really is.

"Do you typically fill out these consent forms or do you have someone else do it?"

"I typically have somebody else witness the signature."

Listen more closely to the question Mo' Dumbest.

"Do you yourself go over the contents as far as the consent form with the patient prior to signing?"

"I do not review word for word the consent form with the patient, no."

"Do you review any aspects of the consent form with the patient?"

"Of this form directly, I do not have this in my hand or refer to it when I'm talking with the patient, no."

Umph-umph-umph! Mo' Dumbest times five.

"Doctor, would you turn to page 28 at the bottom and direct your attention towards the bottom. Do you recognize whose signature that is there?"

"In which?" he asked.

"Witness to signature," Phyllis stated.

"I believe that is Brian Knowles," he said.

"What is his capacity there in the hospital?"

"He's the chief technologist in interventional radiology."

"What is a technologist in interventional radiology; in other words what would his responsibilities be?"

"They assist us during the procedure, their responsibilities are running the x-ray equipment that's utilized, setting up the room prior to procedure, tear down of the room after the procedure, and any other duty we assign during the procedure."

Are you sure you didn't assign Brian to do the procedure, doc? I couldn't have come out any worse if he had.

"Would he have had any knowledge as to UFEs, I mean, how

they are performed and all the information about risks and all that would involve the procedure?"

"I don't believe so, no."

Watch this. Phyllis is moving in for the kill, once again.

"Do you know how long Mr. Knowles has been working there in that location and have you had occasion to work with him at other times?"

"He would have been at Hillside for roughly 20 years."

"Would you have been comfortable with Mr. Brian Knowles describing the UFE procedure with Ms. Kendell including all the risks and all of that?"

"No. I might add we don't expect him to discuss that with the patient. His signature is there present only to confirm that's Ms. Kendell's signature done on that date at that time."

You've just made it clear, doc, that the only important thing for you to do is get my signature on the consent form, not to make sure I completely understand the UFE and all the risks. And that would be a good way to hide the fact that Dr. Langford wasn't going to be the one doing the procedure. Mo' Dumbest times six.

"So you don't have any knowledge as to—you weren't present when this consent form was signed by Ms. Kendell?"

"That's correct."

Bingo again!

Now they're talking about the UFE procedure. I've been waiting to hear this for a long time.

"Isn't it somewhere in the literature that one of the risks of this procedure is that the embolization of the ovaries can also occur and that is one of the reasons that they would not recommend it for women who, you know, want to get pregnant in the future because it could affect the ovaries?" Phyllis asked.

"I believe that is a risk," he said.

"Doctor, could you describe what a Tornado embolization coil is?"

"That's a brand-name, it should have been capitalized, in the vast array of coils that we have available to us. Essentially, all the coils do roughly the same thing. This is a particular design that was made to provide possibly more of an easy embolization using less coils than might normally be required."

I can understand why it would be called a Tornado coil. It tunneled through my uterine arteries and wreaked fatal havoc and destruction on my uterus. Do you mean to tell me you used more than one type of coil?

"I also notice that just below that there is something mentioned as to helical coils, what are those?"

Uh-oh, I jumped the gun. I should have known Phyllis was on to this.

"Helical coils are another design of a similar coil."

"So did you use two different types of coils?"

"Yes."

Lord have mercy! So along with the polyvinyl alcohol particles, you shot an additional two coils up in each of my uterine arteries? No wonder my uterus rotted and died. Instead of putting one rubber band around it, you put two on each side.

Still, Phyllis is not finished.

"Did you use the Tornado and the helical coil on both sides, the left and the right, or one on one side and one on the other side?"

"I believe they were—what was there and stated under the section for right artery embolization, that's what I used in that artery. And then I did a similar procedure possibly using the coil combination on the other side."

"So you used those coils in combination?"

"Yes."

Wow. My perfectly asymptomatic uterus didn't have a chance.

"Is that something that was standard for doctors to do who used the coils in the embolization procedure?"

"There are multiple ways to do a fibroid embolization and this is one of the options that existed at that time for doing fibroid embolization."

Be afraid, ladies. Be very afraid.

"So at the time that you did this procedure using the two coils, you felt that you needed to use two coils instead of one?"

"The number of coils that are used only have bearing in what you're trying to accomplish in the end which is complete cessation of flow in that artery, whatever territory you are embolizing. So, placing one coil or two coils is only in reference to the fact that it took two coils to completely block that artery."

And block it, it did. My poor uterus. It didn't have a chance.

"So what you're saying is that the artery would not have been completely blocked if you had used only the Tornado embolization coil?"

"That is correct."

"So when you did the left uterine artery embolization, you used the same procedure as you did with the right one?"

"Yes, ma'am."

I can't take any more of this. I'm going to have to blink out.

I had to take a break. I'm sorry, but it really got to be too much for me. I knew it was going to be bad but I honestly did not think it would be this bad. I learned through the course of this litigation that coils had been used in addition to the polyvinyl alcohol particles, but this is the first time I heard of *two different types of coils*. In my mind, there is no way my uterus could have survived this complete shut down of the blood supply. And the truth is, it did not. But the pain I endured as my uterus slowly died inside me is beyond description.

When I was told about UFE by the other two doctor-foes, they never ever mentioned anything about any coils being shot up in my uterine arteries. If this was going to happen, I deserved to know it. It is even clearer to me that these bozos did not know what they were talking about. And the pitiful thing is that they didn't know they didn't know because they were too lazy to educate themselves but not too lazy to move full speed ahead to make $7,500.

I lost it there for a few minutes but I'm over it for now. It just makes me even more determined to expose this kind of incompetent medical treatment and stupidity. Let's tune back into the continuing slaughter of Mo' Dumbest by Phyllis.

"Now let me direct your attention to page 58 of Plaintiff's Exhibit Number Five. And Doctor, could you tell me what this document is?" she was asking.

"I believe this is a discharge summary from the hospital that's part of the nurses' notes," he answered.

"So do you recognize the handwriting on this page?"

"I don't recognize the handwriting, no. 21 May 2000, I believe that says 10:20."

That might be what it written, Mo' Dumbest, but I know for a fact I waited all day and well into the afternoon for you to come and discharge me. The nurses were calling you all day with no response. You know, kinda like what happened with Dr. Snyder.

"Now as far as this discharge summary being written, this would have been written with your instructions; is that correct?"

"Yes."

"Down toward the bottom of the page, Doctor, it says follow-up appointment, read what it says there, please, the handwriting?"

"It says: Dr. Rowley will call in, I believe that says two days."

"Did you call Ms. Kendell in two days?"

"Yes."

Now you know you're lying.

"You called her at her home?"

"I returned the call that was placed to me."

See, Mo' Dumbest, you insist on twisting the facts. How could returning a call be the same as making a call? And even the way it's stated, I beg to differ with you. Phyllis is realizing this crap-o-la too.

"You didn't initiate the call, you returned the call, right?"

"Correct."

"But in that telephone call you said you didn't talk with Ms. Kendell, you talked with her mother?"

"Yes, I believe her mother said she was upstairs sleeping."

You mean to tell me my mother called you to tell you I was upstairs sleeping? This is stretching it Mo' Dumbest. Anyway, how is it you remember such details of a little ole phone conversation but on the really important points you "don't recall?" You didn't have an office file on me so I'm sure it's not written down anyplace. How convenient for you to claim you remember this and don't remember so many other important things. Plus, two days after my discharge, I was in so much pain, sleep was no where in my galaxy.

"Did you call back the next day?"

"I did not."

Don't sound so proud about it.

"To speak with Ms. Kendell?"

"No."

Now that sounds like what really happened, bozo.

I see Phyllis is sharpening her knives again. I've learned to read her move-in-for-the-kill body language.

"Doctor, what is your standard protocol as it relates to your follow-up care?" she asked.

I knew it! I knew it!

"That has evolved over the time from when we first started doing these procedures," he said.

Yeah, in other words, you didn't get it right the first time.

"Let's deal with the year 2000 first," Phyllis said.

"There was no set standard protocol that we had for follow-up. We typically give a patient our office phone number so they can get back in contact with us if they had any problems. There was no set method that we all did the same thing," he said.

You're making yourself and your whole radiology group look like real dim-wits, Mo' Dumbest, but I'm happy to see you're telling the truth. But, wait, I don't think you realize what you just said. Mo' Dumbest times seven.

"Did you give Ms. Kendell your telephone number to call?"

"I believe so. I don't know whether that was included with her discharge in the hospital, but she certainly had the number because that was the way that contact had been made previously."

Umph-umph-umph!

"But you didn't specifically say to her here is—"

"No."

"—our phone number for you to call if you have any problems.?"

"Right. I would have done that if I had been able to see her on that Sunday, yes."

I can't resist jumping in right here. You didn't see me on the Sunday of my discharge because you were too busy having a beautiful day to come to the hospital that morning like most doctors do. But, that didn't matter because I had your phone number and I could call you if I wanted to. Still, I don't understand what would have stopped you from calling me that day at home since you missed me at the hospital. Didn't you realize that this was what you should have done since you'd performed my procedure and didn't see me at the time of my discharge? Oh, I get it. This is something new. Discharge-by-phone. Mo' Dumbest times eight.

I'd better pay attention because I see Phyllis is tap-dancing all over his head!

"You are certain you talked with Ms. Kendell's mother?" she asked.

"To the best of my recollection I believe I did," he said.

"So it's possible you didn't?"

This little fire-ball never gives up!

"I either talked to her or Ms. Kendell, but I believe part of the conversation related to when I asked her how she was doing, so I must have been talking to her mother. She said she was upstairs sleeping I think at that time."

Uh-oh, you're having trouble keeping your lies straight. Your stupidity is really out there on this one. Mo' Dumbest times nine.

The little fire-ball is shooting sparks now.

"Now, currently what is your standard protocol as it relates to follow up care for UFE patients?" Phyllis asked.

"Currently I believe the patients are receiving a call I believe within one week after the procedure and follow up phone calls are made at one month, three month and six month," he said.

Three month and six month should be plural, Mo' Dumbest. And this surely didn't happen in my case. Like I said, you guys used me like a cadaver without my authorization. You learned from my maiming and mutilation all the things not to do but, then, didn't have the decency to pass it on to the Fibroid Registry.

"Is there a follow up call made after one week?"

"I believe so."

You don't know? Mo' Dumbest times ten.

"Do you make follow-up calls after one week, Doctor?"

"If the patient would like to talk to me, I will call them, but our nurse practitioner calls them."

If the patient would like to talk to you? You're the one getting paid $7,500 per procedure. Don't you think a little ole phone call should be included in this fee? I hope you're at least splitting fees with the nurse practitioner.

"So what you're saying is the nurse practitioner does call after one week?"

"I believe so."

Oh, Mo' Dumbest, you really don't know, do you? This is really sad.

Now that Phyllis has made it perfectly clear, once again, that Mo' Dumbest doesn't know diddly-squat about what he was doing when he first started performing UFEs, she's satisfied to move on to another topic.

"Doctor, if a UFE patient requires hospitalization post-embolization, do you serve as the attending physician?" she asked.

"No," he said.

"Who does?"

"It's typically the referring physician who sent them to us."

Yeah, like Dr. Snyder who also didn't know diddly-squat.

Watch this. Phyllis is moving in for the kill again. I just love this little fire-ball!

"So if they're having problems as a result of their UFE procedure, you don't readmit them into the hospital, you require that the referring physician does that?"

Told you.

"That's due to an admitting privilege set up where we are allowed to admit for short-term, short-stay admissions, but don't have privilege to admit for an actual direct admission into the hospital that could go on for days."

Like in my case. You mean to tell me you guys didn't even have long-term hospital admitting privileges when you did my UFE? That's pretty cocky isn't it Mo' Dumbest? What if something goes wrong? Excuse me, something did go wrong in my case. Big time. Do you have admitting privileges to the morgue?

"Then what is your understanding of what your role is once the patient is readmitted into the hospital post-embolization?"

Phyllis is off the chain!

"I would assume at that point we become a consultant on the case."

That is, if you can be coaxed out of your hidey-hole.

Pay attention. Phyllis is really taking a walk on the wild side now.

"Doctor, when you say you assume you would become a consultant, are you saying you don't really know, this is the way you think it goes, or what actually does happen?"

LOL! LOL! LOL!

"I'm assuming that we would be alerted to the fact that the patient has been readmitted, but I believe it's only happened one instance so it would be a unique case in that situation."

You were alerted alright, but you still didn't come out of your hidey-hole.

"Do you have any protocols in place for the doctors that perform this procedure as to what your role would be if a patient was readmitted post-embolization?"

I'm going to give you some free advice. Never find yourself on the opposite side of Phyllis Fire-Ball.

"There is no set policy or procedure, no."

Oh-me-gosh! And you fellows had the nerve to solicit for UFE victims? Ladies, I gotta warn you again, be afraid, be very afraid of incompetent doctors. Mo' Dumbest times eleven.

"So each doctor makes the determination as to how they want to deal with that?"

"Each referring doctor, I would say, makes that determination because we ourselves cannot admit them back to the hospital."

Umph-umph-umph! I know I'm on a roll, but I can't help it.

"Is that something that you discuss with the referring doctor at the time that the doctor makes the referral?"

"I don't know. I don't have that conversation with them, no."

Mo' Dumbest times twelve!

Phyllis Fire-Ball is gliding along on roller skates now.

"Do you believe that the Ob/Gyn and the radiologist have to work in collaboration with each other in reference to any post-embolization problems?"

Duh!

"I believe that's at the discretion of the referring physician, but I assume that would be an appropriate thing."

Umph-umph-umph! It's a wrap, another one bites the dust!

Chapter Eleven

The Truth is No Slander

Dr. Rowley's deposition was something else, wasn't it? I have to tell you I really had some rough spots through that one. To have learned that my uterine arteries were shot up with two different types of coils to completely block the blood flow to my uterus was a shocking revelation. When I first heard about the coils being injected into my uterine arteries, along with the polyvinyl alcohol particles, that really upset me. But to discover that there were *two different types of coils* was the zenith of incredulousness.

Now, I'm not overlooking the fact that I am making you endure yet another chapter with me while I face my last demon. I owe you another apology and I'm hopeful you will bear with me for a little longer. I'm sure you'll find that it's worth your time because you will see that this is the granddaddy of all the demons I've had to face.

I'm not going to belabor this point in detail because I would rather that it unfold for you as it will when I take you into the deposition of Dr. Snyder. However, I do think I should make some passing comments about why I think Dr. Snyder deserves his The Dumbest title and the distinction of having a whole chapter in his dis-honor.

Dr. Snyder, as you will recall, was the doc that pushed the button and set all the weapons of body destruction in motion. It was my trust in him that caused me to accept, without question, that what he was saying about UFEs was absolutely the truth, the whole truth and nothing but the truth. Even against the pleading advice of my dear mother whose opinion I respect and hold in high regard.

Dr. Snyder thinks he was the only good guy in this undeniable tragedy. After all, he did come to my rescue and admit me to the hospital after he could not find Dr. Rowley. But the thing he refuses to recognize, which is completely indefensible, is the fact that if he had done his homework and learned the truth about UFEs, he would have known better than to refer me into the unskilled hands of the other doctor-foes. His ignorance and stupidity set everything in motion and, while he may choose to ignore it, I never will. The undeniable truth is, but for him, *none of this would have happened.*

You need to know that Dr. Snyder was dragged to his deposition kicking and screaming. As you will recall, we took the other doctor-foe's depositions in mid-November 2002. We were not able to reel The Dumbest in for his deposition until January 30th, 2003, two and a half months later. But, as you're going to see, it was worth the wait.

Phyllis did not conduct this deposition and, I must say, I was disappointed at first, but Joseph cooked Dr. Snyder on the ole barbie. I'm going to take you, now, into the bowels of this deposition (no pun intended). I'll make sure I keep my mental dialogue going for your edification. Here we go. Dr. Snyder raised his right hand and swore to tell the truth, the same right hand he used to shake my hand and gain my trust to my detriment.

"Now, with regard to uterine fibroid embolization, I take it that's not something that you do in your practice?" Joseph asked.

"I do not do that," Dr. Snyder answered.

"Can you tell me when you first became acquainted with that term or with that procedure; that is, embolization for purposes of treating fibroids? I understand the procedure has been used for other reasons, but uterine fibroid embolization, when did you become familiar with that?"

"I would say that having read about or heard about it through conversations with other physicians that this is beginning to be offered as therapy for some patients. And so prior to me attending the very end of a meeting at the Butler Hospital, I knew that the treatment existed in a nebulous form. In other words, I knew that people were doing this, but I knew not the indications, or the contraindications, and basically only knew that it existed, this treatment existed."

That's not what you told me The Dumbest. From the way you talked, you knew everything under the sun about UFEs. In fact, you did such a good job of convincing me that you knew what you were talking about that the deal was already sealed by the time I talked with Dumbest. I do agree with you on one point: you knew-not-nothing, period. As far as I'm concerned, you knew nothing other than performing hysterectomies at any given occasion.

"All right. You made reference to a fact that there was a meeting at Butler Hospital. Have you had occasion to read Dr. Langford's deposition where he said he conducted a meeting with your group," he asked.

"No, I have not read that," he said.

That's right. You're not big on reading. You're the doc who's never gonna do homework again!

"Okay. Do you recall whether or not that meeting was being overseen or taught by Dr. Langford?"

"No, I don't. And the reason is because I was delivering babies that day. And I had just finished a delivery and went to the department meeting after I delivered the baby, and as I sat down, there was a doctor who was seating himself and I said, 'What did we speak of?' And someone told me; I don't remember who it was, They're wanting, you know, patients for uterine artery embolization. And I said, Oh, okay, well, I'll keep that in mind."

See? I told you they were out culling the field for warm bodies. Weren't there any cadavers available? The way I see it, he had a bounty on my asymptomatic uterus.

"Was it your understanding that either Dr. Langford or somebody from his group was making a presentation to your group?"

"My understanding was that somebody from the radiology department at Butler Hospital was making a presentation to the Ob/Gyn department to make them aware that this is a treatment option that's available for patients in our medical community."

Pay attention to this one.

"Now, I understand your answer with regard to missing the majority of the discussion there. Did you from that point get any additional information about uterine fibroid embolization or the radiology group that was undertaking to perform them; did you hear anything, get some literature?" Joseph asked.

"No. I really didn't. I'm sure that there was a handout that was provided, although I usually don't read those, frequently, so I didn't take one," Dr. Snyder answered.

Unbelievable! This one definitely got his degree from the University of Uterus R Us. The Dumbest times one.

Joseph isn't backing off. He's smooth as an iced-over pond.

"Well, how did you arrive at the decision then or what went into making up your mind to refer a patient to Dr. Langford's group for the purpose of having a uterine fibroid embolization performed on a patient?"

"Based on the fact that going through all of the treatment options that we've briefly discussed earlier today, I didn't really feel like any of them met with any satisfactory—it wasn't a satisfactory care plan for Kellee. She's a busy lady, had a lot of things going on, didn't really have time to be sick but also didn't really have time to have surgery, either. And I believe we met in my Brookford office, which I do not have an ultrasound at, and we decided that we needed to do this pelvic ultrasound to see about the size of the—what we suspicioned were fibroids. And I saw her in the morning."

Well, doc, I wasn't a busy lady anymore once you and the other doctor-foes got through with me. And I know I didn't have time for surgery, but because of you guys, I had to fit multiple surgeries into my schedule. And what's this "we" crap? Weren't you supposed to be the doctor?

Joseph is not letting this bozo off the hook.

"Well, I'm going to get into some detail about that visit and that day, but I'm trying to get before May 15th, 2000, your level of knowledge or familiarity with UFEs, because on that day you talked with her about it. And I'm trying to figure out what did you know and how did you get the information that you did get on UFEs before that day when you first met Kellee?"

Allow me to answer, Joseph. The Dumbest didn't know diddly-squat.

"I already told you that."

Really?

"That was just sitting down and the doctor had made his presentation and you had some general knowledge that it was out there somewhere?"

"Yes."

It gets worse.

"You hadn't done any research or seen any videos or attended any lectures; am I correct?"

"No, that's correct."

I know this is tough to believe but, once again, I'm vindicated. The Dumbest times two.

And still, the unbelievable information keeps coming.

"Okay. And you never spoke with Dr. Langford personally before May 15, 2000, correct?"

"Yeah, that's correct."

"All right. Did you have any understanding as to the risks

associated with UFEs if they were performed on a patient, before May 15th, 2000."

Ooh, this is brutal. I'm really loving this!

"I would say no personal knowledge. I had not reviewed any literature that would give me specific numbers, because being a medical doctor, I—and understanding how the procedure would go, I would be able to surmise where some problems could be. But I have done no personal research and had no knowledge of indications, contraindications or possible complications of the procedure."

"Okay. And specifically, do you know whether it was indicated or contraindicated in patients desiring to maintain her fertility?"

"I had no knowledge of that one way or the other."

Umph-umph-umph!

"Okay. Well, then let's turn to May 15th. Well, let me ask, before we get to that, is that the first date, May 15, 2000, when you first met Kellee Kendell?"

"Yes, that would be the first time we met."

What a tragedy that turned out to be.

"All right. Turn to page four. And under the category abdomen, what does it say there?"

"It says soft, non-tender, and then over to the side I say 18 week fibroid."

"Okay. Is that based on a physical examination that you performed?"

"Yes, sir."

To think I let this incompetent touch me.

"And you were able to palpate a fibroid or fibroids that equaled the size of a uterus that was 18 weeks pregnant?"

"Yes, sir."

"Can fibroids be asymptomatic?

"Absolutely."

Absolutely? But, I guess that asymptomatic fibroids are not lucrative enough.

"Is there any rule of thumb as to whether a particular size fibroid has to be symptomatic or can you have large fibroids and still be asymptomatic?"

"I believe you can have rather large fibroids and be asymptomatic."

Joseph is really getting into the nitty-gritty now.

"Okay. Now, going down to your assessment, if you would, help me understand what you've written there, please."

"It says symptomatic fibroid uterus, check pelvic ultrasound to assess ovaries. Consider Depo Lupron as primary RX treatment. You know, we weren't sure, to the best of my knowledge, that we were going to—if we were going to just try to buy some time by shrinking them down or if we were going to try to go in and do perhaps a myomectomy, because hysterectomy, you know, was out of the question. And, but I knew that we were going to do a one month therapy. And it says as primary RX, or treatment, versus adding a myomectomy. And I say patient given Lupron information."

You're starting with the "we" crap again. I'm glad you remember that hysterectomy was out of the question. Too bad, you didn't take it seriously. Too bad, you allowed me to be violated and didn't value my uterus as much as I did. Or, my life, for that matter.

"Okay. So at that point in time you were considering either Depo Lupron or a myomectomy, but trying to stay away from a myomectomy if Depo Lupron would be effective?"

"I think at that point in my mind I wanted to do what I could to help diminish her symptoms and give her time to make a decision on whether she wanted to take time out from her busy schedule to have a myomectomy or, you know, proceed perhaps with six months of therapy versus three months and see if the uterus wouldn't stay small long enough to allow her to get things in order. So at that point when I wrote that note, when I was writing that note, the first step was trying to decrease her symptoms, and the second step would be determined at a later date after we reviewed the therapy."

What symptoms are you talking about The Dumbest? The fact that I had a fibroid uterus? Because I wasn't having in symptoms from my fibroids and you know it.

"Okay. Now, you started to give me answers earlier on about whether or not—you said that you didn't have the ultrasound machine at your office and therefore you had to send her someplace. Where did she go?"

"To our main office which is in Fairburn."

"And do you call ahead or have somebody call ahead and say she's on the way?"

"Basically we'll just call down and I tell my ultrasound tech that I would like for her to have an ultrasound today rather than waiting, and so we ask that she have the ultrasound done. So she was sent that very day. And I believe I was seeing patients that afternoon in Fairburn, so when I arrived in Fairburn the ultrasounding was just being completed and so I had the benefit of reviewing that with Miss Kendell at that time."

"Okay. Was the ultrasound of assistance to you, first of all, in determining whether you're dealing with a fibroid or a cancerous tumor?"

"It—yes, it was."

"What did it tell you?"

"It told me that the, first of all, that the ovaries appeared to be normal; it also showed me that there was no ascites fluid, and it also showed me that the texture of the uterus was and the fibroids was of an echogenicity that would be consistent with a fibroid, benign tumor."

"Okay. Since you began your conversation with Kellee Kendell concerning Depo Lupron at your Farmington office, did you continue that conversation then in your Fairburn office?"

Now we're getting to it.

"Yes, I did have the opportunity to do that."

"Just describe for me, as best you can recall it, how that conversation went and what was the decision made."

"We reviewed the findings and decided at that point to go

ahead and do the Depo Lupron as we had decided. I gave her some samples of some medication to help with the side effect of hot flashes. And the best that I remember—as I recall, I still just felt like this was not the treatment that she was looking for; it did not fit with what was going on in her life. And as she was actually leaving I remembered my—I remembered that there were radiologists that had privileges at Butler Hospital that were interested in interviewing patients like her. So as she was leaving I believe I kind of intercepted her on the way out the door and I said that this is another treatment option, would you be interested in hearing from these doctors, does this sound like something that you would be interested in? And she answered in the affirmative so then I went about contacting the radiology department and asked them to put me with whoever—whichever physician it was that would do these types of procedures."

The Dumbest times four. Did they toss a coin or draw straws? This was clearly a CYA response. Why did I need further treatment for asymptomatic fibroids? This really really ticks me off. The Dumbest is trying to make it sound like he just innocently raised this question to me and left everything up to me, like he did my recovery. And, anyway, does it make sense to give a patient a Depo Lupron shot as the treatment and then say, "Oh, by the by, now that I've just stuck you in your butt, I've thought of something else that might work for you?" I clearly remember that The Dumbest did not call me until the next day. Remember, his memory is affected by what he needs to say to save his butt. It's really not clever at all.

Joseph is switching tactics.

"All right. Now, did you have any understanding at this time as to her desire to maintain her fertility?" Joseph asked.

"Yes, I knew that a hysterectomy was not an option for her," Dr. Snyder replied.

Will wonders never cease?

"Was she fairly insistent or convincing that this was something that she absolutely wanted to have, she wanted to preserve her fertility? Did she impress upon you the importance of this to her?"

"Yeah, I knew that—I knew that that was her desire."

You knew it was my desire but it wasn't important to you. As soon as you got me in trouble, the first thing you wanted to do was hide your mess by cutting my uterus out. So no, it wasn't important to you.

"Okay. Now, as you've described it, you said that at some point it occurred to you that there's another modality of uterine fibroid embolization that you had heard about or had come acquainted with, and you raised that as a prospect with Kellee as she was leaving the office; is that the way it worked?"

That's right. Stick it to him Joseph.

"Yes. That's my recollection."

But it's not my recollection.

"Okay. Tell me what, if anything, you can recall telling her that time with regard to what it is and what it can accomplish and what she can expect from it."

I'm all ears.

"I believe that I would have related to her that it was a nonsurgical way to shrink fibroids without the use of medications and without the—and that it would preserve her uterus."

The Dumbest, you're moving closer to the truth. Of course the truth is a lot easier to remember, isn't it?

"Given the limited amount of knowledge that you had about that procedure, could you be very specific with her as to how — the technique by which it's done—

"No."

"The side effects, the recuperation period and all of that?"

"No. I would just know that it was inserted through a blood vessel, you know, and likely in the groin is what I assumed, and that it would selectively—the radiologist would selectively try to go up the uterine artery and block it so that the—so that the blood supply to the uterus and therefore the fibroids is diminished. So that the fibroids basically sort of lose nutrition and start to wither on their own."

Well, The Dumbest, what I know is that you told me about UFEs in a way that left no doubt in my mind that you completely and absolutely knew what you were talking about. As I've said many times, you did such a good job that the deal was sealed by the time I called Dr. Langford. Don't you remember the script after rehearsal? Simple 24-hour out patient procedure?

Joseph isn't backing off.

"This is something that you probably knew and therefore communicated to her on May 15th?"

"I would say that I would have described—that would be the extent of my knowledge, and I would have tried to relate to her the basic premise of the procedure without knowledge of whether she was a good candidate or not, without knowledge of, you know, risks, benefits, that sort of stuff. I knew that it was a—a treatment that existed and I wanted to know if she thought it would—would it be at least of interest to her such that I might share her history with another doctor and get his opinion."

You'd better watch it, The Dumbest. Your stories aren't adding up. You mean you told me all this while I was on the way out the door? I don't think so. It happened just as I've stated it. You called me the next day and told me you had discussed my case with Dr. Langford and you described the UFE in detail. After you convinced me I was a prime candidate you informed me that Dr. Langford was expecting my call. At this time, I had been successfully reeled in.

The Dumbest times five.

"Did you specifically ask for Dr. Langford or did you ask for somebody in that practice that was knowledgeable?" Joseph asked.

"I asked for somebody in the practice that was knowledgeable and that was performing the procedure," Dr. Snyder answered.

You were calling the wrong number for that.

"Okay. And not having any prior experience with Dr.

Langford, your knowledge of his background, competence, whatever, take me through that conversation and what you learned and what he told you."

"First of all, that he had privileges at the hospital and that he had been doing procedures there, I felt that he was a reasonable person to speak to regarding any said procedure. I would have related to him Kellee's age, the number of children that she's had and the size of the uterus based on the ultrasound examination that I gave to him, and I would have reviewed likely her symptoms and her desire not to have a hysterectomy or an invasive surgery. And at that point, then I would have asked him did he feel that she would be a reasonable candidate for the procedure that he would provide."

This response is just chock-full of all kind of goodies. It looks good at first blush, but closer inspection reveals a myriad of flaws. First of all, Dr. Langford had never done a UFE. Second, if Dr. Langford had a modicum of understanding about UFEs, he would have known I was not a prime candidate for two glaringly obvious reasons: 1) My desire not to have a hysterectomy and, 2) My desire not to have invasive surgery.

"Okay. Before I get to his response to you, did you communicate to him her desire to maintain her fertility?"

"I communicated to him that she did not want to have a hysterectomy. I do not remember if I told him she wants to have more babies. But one would assume that that's why she wanted to keep the uterus."

Very good. I would not have expected you to make this mammoth deduction.

"Okay. So other than reviewing then her pertinent gynecologic history and her ultrasound findings, you asked him then whether she was a fit candidate for this procedure?

"Yes."

"And tell me what his response was, what you learned from him."

I can't wait to hear this.

"He, to my knowledge, or to my recollection, he answered in the affirmative that she would be a person that could consider it as a treatment option, but he did not go over why. So in other words, he didn't tell me if there was a size that was too big or too small or anything other than based on what I told him he thought that she might be a reasonable person to check it out, to see if that's what she might want to do. So that's the gist of the conversation."

"Okay. Did he ask you to send him your medical records so that he could review them before making a decision about whether she was an appropriate candidate?"

This would have been wise, but I doubt he bothered to do this.

"I don't remember."

Umph-umph-umph!

"Did he communicate to you any more about the specifics of UFEs and how they were performed?"

"No."

You didn't ask? The Dumbest times six.

"Did he tell you about the recuperation period, how many hours, days, weeks it would take to recover?"

I've been waiting for this one.

"I believe he may have told me that, you know, the procedure is done and then patients frequently stay overnight in the hospital, maybe one or two days, and receive medication, pain medication through the IV, because there is a bit of pain associated with it right at the beginning. But that would be the extent of it. And of course some of this I've learned since in trying to further assist Miss Kendell in her access to health care, and so it's hard for me to remember exactly when I learned that part of the equation."

The first part of your response was closer to the truth. And the "a bit of pain" part sounds about right because if I had known anything about the pain from hell associated with UFEs, I know I would never have agreed to it. The last part is debatable. You didn't bust a book in trying to learn more about UFEs in assisting me in my access to health care.

Watch this. Joseph's getting ready to slice and dice him.

"Okay. I appreciate that. Trying as best you can to isolate the information he gave you at that point, because you're going to take this information and communicate it to Kellee Kendell, did he in any way put a time frame within which she should be able to go back to work?"

"No. I don't—I do not remember that."

Well, I remember. I was supposed to have the UFE on Friday and be back to work on Monday.

"Did he discuss with you his success rate as far as doing these procedures?"

"No."

Again, you didn't ask? The Dumbest times seven.

"Did he tell you anything about his personal experience in performing these procedures?"

"No."

Again, you didn't ask. The Dumbest times eight.

"Was it important to you before you sent Kellee Kendell to him to ascertain whether or not he had knowledge or experience in this?"

You're kicking butt now Joseph!

"Of course it's very important to a physician, if he sends someone to another physician in consultation, then that person be a qualified physician. And by virtue of him practicing at Butler Hospital and having privileges there, I believe that it's a good radiology department for them to discuss risks, benefits, contraindications and for them to help her decide whether this was the right procedure for her."

So where were they going to discuss this with me? In the tent set up in the parking lot? Do you really believe this is enough when you're talking about putting a person's life in the hands of another doctor?

The Dumbest times nine.

Joseph is not letting him off the hook.

"You didn't explore with him his personal background,

knowledge or experience in the performance of UFEs, during that conversation; is that correct?"

"I did not."

This is so good.

"That's correct, correct?"

"That is correct, I did not explore his personal—

Umph-umph-umph!

"All right. Now, did he volunteer to you that this was a new procedure that he and his group were just undertaking to perform?"

"I knew that it was a new procedure for the hospital, so—but I had no knowledge of how many prior procedures had been done. I know that this is a—this type of procedure has been done for many years, but usually in the context of bleeding more so than actually trying to treat fibroids. And so it's just the same procedure with a different indication. And so—but no, I made no attempt to ascertain the number or how long they had been doing it for this indication."

Tripped over your tongue a bit didn't you, doc? Your brain had a hard time making your tongue say something so ridiculous.

The Dumbest times ten.

Joseph has turned into hot ice now.

"All right. If you were unconvinced as to his competence and knowledge in the area, would you have been reluctant to refer Kellee to them?"

"Absolutely."

Kur-plunk! He fell right into that trap. The Dumbest times eleven.

"Okay. Now, did you and Dr. Langford discuss the administration of Depo Lupron to Kellee Kendell or the one—the shot that you had just given her a day or two before?"

"I believe that we did."

"And tell me about what—how that transpired, what was discussed and what he said?"

"I basically said I've just given her a shot of Depo Lupron to help shrink her fibroids; do you think that that would potentially be a problem? And I believe that he felt that it would not potentially be a problem. Because they're both—in my thought, the reason why I did not believe it to be a potential problem was because they're both trying to achieve the same thing, perhaps by slightly different mechanisms. But the goal is to basically starve off the fibroid through removal of hormonal support and, with that, decreasing blood flow, and then his procedure would mechanically decrease blood flow. So, you know, they could be considered complementary, although there certainly aren't any studies that would suggest that that's how things should be done."

Slightly different mechanisms? One's a little ole shot in my butt and the other is an incision in my groin and then tubing is stuck up into my uterine arteries. Then polyvinyl alcohol particles were shot through the tubing along with two sets of coils. And you call this "slightly different mechanisms?" And remember, The Dumbest, you don't read so how would you know anything about the studies? But you know plenty about the recommendation of hysterectomies for your patients.

The Dumbest times twelve.

"Do you know of any information, any studies that have been done where a patient has undergone a UFE after having received a Depo Lupron shot?"

"I do not."

See? I told you.

"Okay. Do you have a medical opinion as to whether or not the prior administration of Depo Lupron would potentiate the effect of a UFE and its mechanical occlusion of the vascular supply to the fibroid?"

"I don't have a medical opinion on that."

Oh, but you should have before you turned me over into the hands of the incompetence of the other doctor-foes.

"Okay. Now, after this conversation with Dr. Langford, did you then communicate or call or talk with Kellee Kendell?"

"I believe that I did, yes. I called her."

"You initiated the conversation. And tell me how that conversation went."

"Would be that I discussed her case with the radiologist and that I felt that—that he indicated to me that she would be a reasonable candidate, and I gave her his phone number that I had marked in the chart there."

There was a lot more than that involved. You sealed the deal.

"Okay. Did you communicate to her what he said to you about the mechanism of the procedure and the number of days in the hospital and the pain medication she's going to get and the discomfort level during the first few days? Did you get into that much detail with her?"

Pow-pow-pow!

"I don't recall, but I would have tried to, I think. If I had anything to offer her, I would have tried. My nature is to do that. But I do not recall."

You did a lot more than tried.

Watch this. Joseph comes in through the back door and whacks him.

"Okay. I forgot to ask you, but during the conversation you had with Dr. Langford, did you and he discuss who is going to follow the patient after the procedure?"

"No, sir."

"Did you have any understanding of what would happen if post-procedure care was needed?"

"No, I did not."

The Dumbest times thirteen.

"Okay. At that time, if the question had been asked of you— Who's going to take care of Kellee Kendell after the procedure?—what would have been your expectation."

"My expectation would be the person who performed the procedure would care for them afterwards."

Joseph is changing direction.

"Did you have any knowledge while she was in the hospital

as to whether or not Dr. Langford or some other doctor was going to actually do the procedure?" he asked.

"No," Dr. Snyder answered.

"Did you ever get a letter or other communication from them, as is common from one doctor to another, telling you that they had just done a procedure on your patient and summarizing what they did and what they found?"

"No."

"Did they call you after she was discharged to tell you that they had done this procedure and tell you what they did?"

"No."

"Isn't it common for doctors to provide that kind of information to the patient's primary care physician?"

"As a courtesy, yes. It would not be uncommon to do that."

"But you never heard from them with regard to the specifics of what they found and what they did in this procedure?"

"That is correct."

"Now, you've had an opportunity to look at the procedure note and to review the specifics of the manner in which Dr. Rowley performed the UFE. Do you have—"

"Excuse me. I have not," Dr. Snyder interjected.

"Even to this day?"

"Even to this day I have not looked at this procedure, no. There was no note furnished to my medical records."

Is this not incredible? The Dumbest times fourteen.

"Okay."

"And this is the first time that I've seen this," Dr. Snyder said.

"Okay. I thought maybe it had come to you in the course of the litigation."

"No. No, sir."

This kind of lack of concern and interest is just plain indifferent and lazy. I guess it's hard to study and hide at the same time.

"Okay. Once again I'll ask you the question, what would have been your expectation with regard to follow up care for symptoms or problems associated with the performance of the UFE; that is, you or the doctor who did the procedure?"

"I would assume that the doctor who did the procedure would be the one that would do the aftercare and help manage—and manage any possible complications from the procedure."

It would have been a really good idea for you guys to have discussed this in advance. You know what happens when you assume. Just like you assumed I was a prime candidate but knew nothing about the procedure.

Joseph is moving to a different issue.

"Then the next message, or the next time that I see anything would be May 25, would be the left side of the same page, and do you recall that communication?" he asked.

"I recall that the communication was made, yes," he answered.

"Okay. Tell me as best you can, after reviewing that note, what was communicated to you and what decision you made?"

"Basically that Kellee's mother was in her attendance and that she was in unbearable pain and getting worse instead of better and wants us to help her and thinks maybe she should be placed back in the hospital."

It was the pain from hell.

"Okay. I take it then that the—as best you can reconstruct it from that note, you didn't personally speak with Kellee before she made it to the hospital?

"As best that I can reconstruct, that would be fair."

I'm going to bring you in on another area of interest.

"Obviously this note reflects that you now know that Dr. Rowley has done the procedure, correct?" Joseph asked.

"Yes," Dr. Snyder answered.

"Okay. Did it concern you at all or was it of importance to you that you spoke with Dr. Langford, you communicated with Dr. Langford, Dr. Langford seemed to be competent based upon your initial communications with him, and then here's Dr. Rowley having done the procedure, a person you didn't know?"

"I would say that usually the way my practice works is that if you've made contact with—a patient has made contact with you regarding a certain procedure, then you've established a relationship with that person, and that's who the patient plans on doing the procedure. So in other words, one of my patients wouldn't necessarily expect to see somebody else on the day of their hysterectomy, they would expect to see me."

Odd you should use hysterectomy as an example. Sounds like you really like those.

"In Kellee's position, having communicated with Dr. Langford, would you have anticipated that Dr. Langford would be the person who would do the UFE?"

"Yes, I would."

You bet I would.

"Okay. Do you know Dr. Rowley?"

"No."

"Had you ever communicated with him at any point about his competence and experience and background and training in UFEs.?"

"No."

"All right. And did you have any understanding as to the magnitude of the pain that she would be experiencing so as to determine whether or not—a pain greater than a ten is not supposed to be possible, but..."

"Worst pain she's ever experienced."

You got that right.

"Okay. Do you have any understanding as to whether or not that would be a normal and expected side effect, from the conversations that you had with Dr. Langford?"

"From my conversations and the general understanding, I believed that patients would not have that much discomfort from that procedure."

For once, we agree.

"Okay. Turning to page 18 in Exhibit Number 1, which is your office record. There's a note in your office record that is dated June 15th, 2000. Do you recall whether or not you had any communications with Kellee or her mother between May 28th and June 15th?"

"I don't recall."

"And from looking at this note, is this a note which would reflect the fact that she came into your office for evaluation?"

"For follow up, yes."

"Take me through the evaluation and what you found."

"Three and a half weeks status post uterine artery embolization complicated by post-op readmission. Possible infection in ileus, I write, and no fevers, meaning currently. No GI symptoms, currently. Occasional spotting, which would revert to vaginal bleeding. Still having waves of pain. Cannot lift. Pain on top on left very sharp."

"Okay. What was your plan?" Joseph asked.

I'd like an answer to this too, doc.

"At that point I said one month status post uterine artery embolization with apparent early failure. Uterus near 20 week size, in parentheses 18 weeks by my prior exam. Check pelvic ultrasound to confirm size and will discuss with interventional radiology. Patient is understandably very upset." Dr. Snyder answered.

Oh, yes. I was really upset. I was still having severe pain a month later and I was told I would have some discomfort for two days after the procedure.

"Between May 28th and June 15th, had you made any efforts to contact Dr. Rowley or any member of the interventional radiology group?"

"I don't recall. Prior to—it seems like that I did try to contact them a couple of times after seeing Kellee, just because I wanted to know what their opinion was. But I honestly—last I really knew they were following her in the hospital and I, you know, believed that they would continue to follow her as an outpatient after the procedure, knowing that there was a problem with the procedure."

Tried to contact them a couple of times? You know you're lying through your teeth. Oh, I get it. You've got to cover for the other doctor-foes because all of you have the same medical malpractice insurance carrier.

"How do you go about or who would you call to try to communicate with Dr. Rowley?"

"I would go to—I would have went back to the number that I recorded in the chart, on the ultrasound report, which would have been the radiology department, because there's no real office where they see patients and examine patients. So there's no good central area of contact. They don't give out pagers, so my only option was to—pager numbers, so my only option was to call and leave messages with—with who, I don't know."

Umph-umph-umph! You kinda stumbled on that one, doc. If you knew Dumbest and Mo' Dumbest didn't have a real office, why would you send me to them?

The Dumbest times fifteen.

"Okay. And in response to those messages that you left, you didn't get a call back from any member of the group?"

"I do not remember getting any calls back."

"Did you ever communicate to Kellee that if I don't hear from them I'm going to go over to the hospital and find him?"

"It's a possibility, yeah."

"Okay. Did you have an understanding from her that she was led to believe that this was going to be a 48-hour deal, where she'd have pain and she'd be able to go about her normal life?"

"That's my understanding."

"Okay. Did you at any time finally manage to speak with Dr. Rowley and what were the circumstances of that?"

"I don't remember any further discussions."

Yes you do.

"Okay. There was a reference I heard from somebody, and maybe you can help me understand, that Dr. Rowley had communicated that it wasn't uncommon for pain and discomfort to continue for a period up to six months. Do you remember ever receiving that report from Dr. Rowley or somebody?"

"Or somebody. It's possible. It's possible."

It's more than possible. It's the reason I walked around for six months with my uterus rotting inside me.

"Okay. Do you recall what her reaction was if you did in fact communicate that to her?"

"Yeah, it seems like that perhaps I did, now, that there was some kind of communication and that it seems like that she was a little bit distraught because she was under the impression that she didn't realize it was going to take that long for her to get better. So I do remember that now."

This was the most serious mistake you docs made and you had trouble remembering it?

The Dumbest times sixteen.

"Do you recall when it was that you became aware that she was in Burton Hospital?"

"It seems like that Dr. Thomas has associates, fellows, people that he trains, and I believe that when she was admitted to the hospital they called me and told me that she was there and they were caring for her."

They were doing more than caring for me, The Dumbest. They were in a fight to save my life.

"Were you asked to come over and see her or participate in her care at all?

"No."

Oh, yes. I remember this one well. You "declined" to come to Burton Hospital.

"Okay. Do you have an explanation, an opinion yourself as to why Kellee had the problems that were discovered in November of 2000?"

"I would assume that during the course of the procedure that some way the bowel had become compromised, and whether—

and by what exact mechanism I know not what. But retrospectively one would think that something compromised the bowel, in which she developed all these symptoms for. Perhaps putting her in the hospital, giving her IV fluids and antibiotics sort of cooled things off enough that she was able to leave the hospital, but that there still was an ongoing problem and that it ultimately came to a head again, and she, I believe, went to Burton emergency department and that's how she ended up in the hospital."

It's amazing how screwed up you can get things. By the way, I was rushed to the hospital in an ambulance. I didn't just casually walk into Burton's emergency department.

Now this next question takes the cake and is a good note to close the door on.

"Have you done any research with regard to Kellee Kendell's — the issues in Kellee Kendell's care and treatment?"

"No, I have not."

The Dumbest times seventeen.

See, I told you this one was never gonna do homework again!

※ ※ ※

This is not a court of Justice young man, this is a court of Law.
—Oliver Wendell Holmes

This is a true story. I have told the truth, the whole truth and nothing but the truth. I know it may be hard for some readers to believe that the events as stated in this book, actually happened. Often, it was hard for me to believe it happened. So many times, I have wished, with all my heart, that all this never happened to me. I have wished that I could turn back the hands of time to May 2000 and play out my life in an entirely different manner.

I would not have wished this mis-experience on anybody

including the doctors that performed the negligent acts. I surely would have deleted the whole medical catastrophe as though it never happened. But unfortunately it did. I will never get my uterus back no matter how much I grieve the loss of it. I will never be able to erase the thoughts I have of the violation of my body which I deem to be equivalent to being assaulted. I give this comparison because Dr. Rowley touched my body without my authorization. I was not informed that he would inject foreign objects into my uterine arteries that would cause me to be maimed and almost caused my death. I will never be able to erase the ugly scar on my abdomen that I am forced to wear everyday for the rest of my life as an unwelcome reminder of the overwhelming betrayal I suffered at the hands of the three doctors depicted throughout this book. I feel as though I have been branded.

Throughout my part in writing this book, I had to pray for the strength to willingly relive every painful moment that I suffered for over three years. It was not an easy task. The havoc wreaked on my emotions took an incredible toll on my body, mind, and spirit.

I derived strength from the determination that I would tell my true story about my UFE in the hope that I would save other women from suffering my grim fate. I derived strength from the determination that as long as there was breath in my body, I would not stop until this kind of medical treachery was revealed. And even if I died, I believed that Phyllis knew I would not rest easy in my grave if she did not tell my story for me. We both shared the same passionate outrage for what happened to me, and what might possibly be happening to other women with fibroids.

Be afraid of the fact that very little research has gone into determining the long term effects of this procedure. Be aware, that some doctors are not telling the whole truth about uterine fibroid embolization in terms of the risks and potential complications. I will never believe that my case is an isolated incident. Even though it is true that many women have benefited from this procedure, the potential is out there for many women to be harmed if they are unlucky enough, as I was, to fall into the hands of incompetent doctors.

I have always heard of the Hippocratic Oath, that is the oath that all physicians swear to upon becoming medical doctors. All through this travesty of medical treatment, I kept questioning whether the Hippocratic Oath was still in existence or a thing of the past. I was so consumed by this question that I decided to revisit the Hippocratic Oath and share it with you. It confirmed what I had been raised to believe all along, and that is that doctors are bound by the oath to take care of and protect their so trusting patients. I will allow you to read it and judge for yourself whether this was true in my case or not.

Hippocratic Oath

I swear to fulfill, to the best of my ability and judgment, this covenant:

I will respect the hard-won scientific gains of those physicians in whose steps I walk, and gladly share such knowledge as is mine with those who are to follow.

I will apply, for the benefit of the sick, all measures which are required, avoiding those twin traps of overtreatment and therapeutic nihilism.

I will remember that there is art to medicine as well as science, and that warmth, sympathy, and understanding may outweigh the surgeon's knife or the chemist's drug.

I will not be ashamed to say "I know not," nor will I fail to call in my colleagues when the skills of another are needed for a patient's recovery.

I will respect the privacy of my patients, for their problems are not disclosed to me that the world may know. Most especially must I tread with care in matters of life and death. If it is given to me to save a life, all thanks. But it may also be within my power to take a life; this awesome responsibility must be faced with great humbleness and awareness of my own frailty. Above all, I must not play at God.

I will remember that I do not treat a fever chart, a cancerous growth, but a sick human being, whose illness may affect the person's family and economic stability. My responsibility includes these related problems, if I am to care adequately for the sick.

I will prevent disease whenever I can, for prevention is preferable to cure.

I will remember that I remain a member of society, with special obligations to all my fellow human beings, those sound of mind and body as well as the infirm.

If I do not violate this oath, may I enjoy life and art, respected while I live and remembered with affection thereafter. May I always act so as to preserve the finest traditions of my calling and may I long experience the joy of healing those who seek my help.

Written in 1964 by Louis Lasagna, Academic Dean of the School of Medicine at Tufts University, and used in many medical schools today.

Epilogue

Georgia December 2003

The moon-filtered bedroom was dark and silent as my eyes flew open in panic and alarm. I had been jerked awake as the familiar knife-like pain centered on my navel and shot through my abdomen. I closed my eyes tightly as I said a soundless and fervent prayer. Please God, don't let this be happening to me again.

But the pain was undeniable and the well-known sensations throughout my body were like unwanted demons returned to haunt me, once again. I lay perfectly still, knowing that any movement would precipitate the wretched vomiting. I was hoping against hope that I was still asleep and somehow trapped in a nightmare from which I would awaken any moment.

It was no use. I bolted from my bed as the unmistakable bile rose with frightening rapidity into my throat and threatened to project from my mouth before I could make it to the bathroom. I slid onto the floor in front of the commode where I emptied the contents of my stomach in painful and projectile torrents that caused me to be incontinent. As always, with these episodes, the vomiting came in intervals which forced me to lie on the bathroom floor as I waited for the next attack.

The murky light of dawn was trickling through the bedroom blinds as I walked weakly to my bed and climbed back in. A glance at the clock told me it was 6:00 a.m. Was it possible that I was in the bathroom for three hours? I had lost track of time as I lay on the hard cold bathroom tiles. Once back in bed, I was too nauseous to do anything but lie in a fetal position as I prayed for this episode to pass. For the first time during one of these attacks, I was alone and without help. I was frightened.

I refused to accept that this was happening to me again. I was so close to the year-mark since I had my last episode. My doctor told me that if I could go a year without another attack, the worst might be over and I might stop having bowel obstructions. This was too cruel. In two more weeks, I would have reached the anniversary of my last attack, and now this. I did not want to think the inevitable because that might give life to my fears. I lay still and silent as I willed my body to not betray me by presenting me with another bowel obstruction that could lead to another dreaded surgery or death.

By 10:00 a.m. the pain was coming in waves and I had made several more trips to the bathroom where I retched and brought up vile green bile as there was no longer anything left in my stomach. I was no longer able to deny what was happening and I became morbidly afraid that any moment my organs would shut down. I rolled over and reached for the phone and called the one person I knew would come to my aid, but more important, who would fiercely protect me and not allow anyone to let me die. Phyllis.

With relief, I heard her voice as she answered her phone on the other end of the line.

"Phyllis," I said in a small weak voice, "I've been vomiting all night."

After asking me a series of questions, in rapid-fire order she said, "I'm on my way…"